# THE FUTURE OF NURSING EDUCATION

## AN INTERNATIONAL UTSTEIN REPORT

National League for Nursing

# THE FUTURE OF NURSING EDUCATION

## AN INTERNATIONAL UTSTEIN REPORT

*Edited by*

**Gordon Lee Gillespie,** PhD, DNP, RN, ANEF, FAAN

**Sandra Davis,** PhD, DPM, ACNP-BC, FAANP, FAAN

**Beverly Malone,** PhD, RN, FAAN

Wolters Kluwer

Philadelphia • Baltimore • New York • London
Buenos Aires • Hong Kong • Sydney • Tokyo

*Acquisitions Editor:* Heather Bays-Petrovic
*Senior Development Editor:* Emily Schlapp
*Marketing Manager:* Amy Whitaker
*Production Project Manager:* Kirstin Johnson
*Manager, Graphic Arts & Design:* Stephen Druding
*Manufacturing Coordinator:* Margie Orzech
*Prepress Vendor:* S4Carlisle Publishing Services



9 8 7 6 5 4 3 2 1

Printed in the United States of America

---

**Library of Congress Cataloging-in-Publication Data**

ISBN-13: 978-1-975282-13-4

Library of Congress Control Number: 2026941643

---



shop.lww.com

WALS0626

# About the Authors

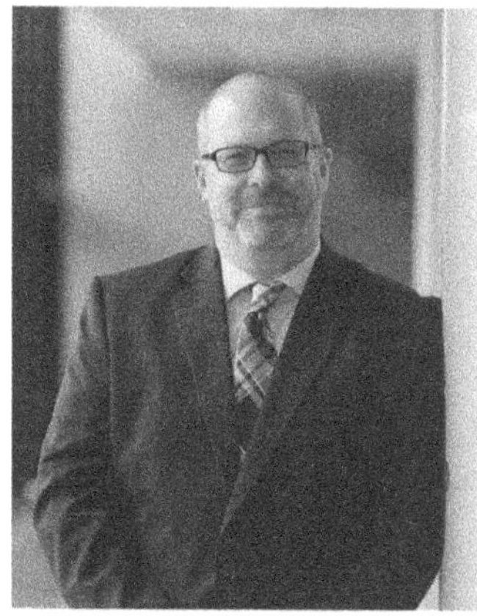

**Gordon Lee Gillespie**, PhD, DNP, RN, CEN, CNE, CPEN, PHCNS-BC, ANEF, FAEN, FAAN, has been a registered nurse for 30 years working in emergency department, public health, and academic settings. Dr. Gillespie's research on workplace violence against health care workers has been funded by the U.S. CDC-National Institute for Occupational Safety and Health (NIOSH), Robert Wood Johnson Foundation, American Nurses Foundation, and Emergency Nurses Association Foundation. Dr. Gillespie has been invited by the CDC-NIOSH to develop an educational program on workplace bullying and consult on two national online learning modules. His work has been cited by the U.S. Occupational Safety and Health Administration, U.S. Government Accountability Office, American Nurses Association (ANA), and by practitioners and researchers across five continents. He chaired the national workplace violence conference, guest edited two interprofessional journal issues on workplace violence, co-chaired the Registered Nurses' Association of Ontario's second edition of the Best Practice Guideline "Preventing and Managing Bullying and Violence in the Workplace," and served as an international director of the Emergency Nurses Association. Dr. Gillespie also serves on the National Academies of Sciences, Engineering, and Medicine's Forum to Address Attacks on Health Professionals. In 2024, Dr. Gillespie received the Lifetime Achievement Award from the Emergency Nurses Association. Currently, Dr. Gillespie is the chief program officer for the National League for Nursing (NLN) and an adjunct professor at the University of Cincinnati College of Nursing.

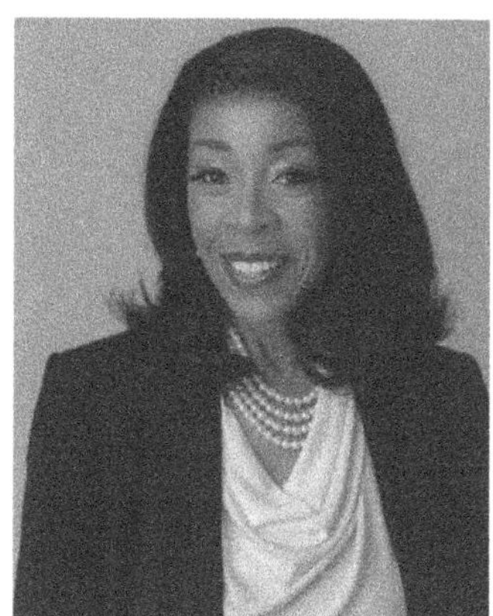

**Sandra Davis**, PhD, DPM, ACNP-BC, FAANP, FAAN, is an accomplished nurse leader with decades of experience in academia and practice. Having served in faculty, administrative, clinical practice, and leadership roles, Dr. Davis brings depth, breadth, and passion to her work. Currently, Dr. Davis is deputy chief director for the NLN/Walden University College of Nursing Institute for Social Determinants of Health and Social Change. Now in its fourth cohort, the Institute is equipping nurse educators and interprofessional colleagues with leadership competencies to integrate social determinants of health into programs and curricula and publish with broad dissemination. In addition, Dr. Davis chairs the International Council of Nurses (ICN) Education Experts Advisory Committee where she brings her knowledge and experience to broadening the commitment to quality and equity in nursing education around the world. Prior to joining the NLN, Dr. Davis was associate professor and inaugural associate dean for diversity, equity, and inclusion at the George Washington University School of Nursing. Her research and scholarly interests include health inequities, social and structural determinants of health, structural competency, and antiracism. She was the principal investigator on a participatory action photovoice project, *The Social Determinants of a Heart Healthy Community*, that was exhibited at the Smithsonian National Museum of African American History and Culture in Washington, D.C. Dr. Davis is an award-winning author who most recently co-edited the book *Nurse Leaders Driving Health Equity: Tackling Social and Structural Determinants* and co-authored the article "Introducing the 'Nursing Education Integrating Social Change for Health Equity (NISCHE)' Framework for Nursing Education." Dr. Davis is a board-certified acute-care nurse practitioner and past president of the Nurse Practitioner Association of the District of Columbia. She holds multiple fellowships and is the recipient of numerous awards and distinctions.

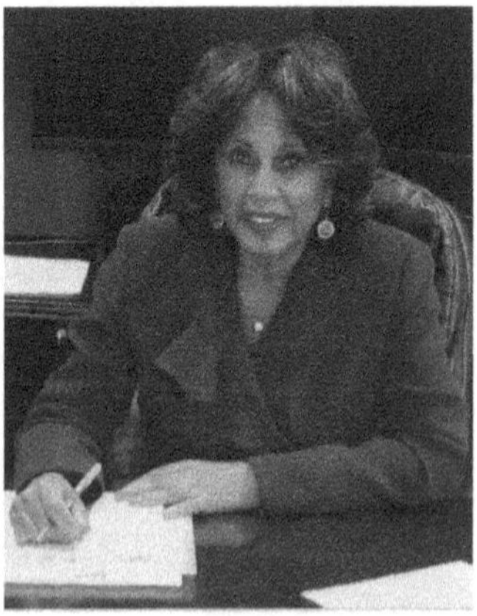

**Beverly Malone**, PhD, RN, FAAN, is a health care leader, accomplished innovator, and nursing champion. Under her leadership, the NLN has advanced the science of nursing education through enhancing stakeholder collaboration, increasing diversity in nursing scholarship, and championing evidence-based practice. Dr. Malone's distinguished career has blended policy, education, administration, and clinical practice, including serving as federal deputy assistant secretary for health under President Bill Clinton. As a reviewer, she contributed to the groundbreaking Institute of Medicine report, *The Future of Nursing: Leading Change, Advancing Health*, and served on the Minority Health Federal Advisory Committee. Dr. Malone has been awarded more than 20 honorary doctorates. Presently, Dr. Malone serves as vice chair at the Institute for Healthcare Improvement Board of Directors, co-leads the National Academy of Medicine (NAM) Health Professional Education and Communication Working Group, and serves on NAM's Steering Committee. She is also a member of ecoAmerica's Leadership Circle Executive Committee. She has received numerous awards including 2024 Hall of Fame Award from the ANA; Mary Elizabeth Carnegie Leadership in Equity, Diversity, and Inclusivity Award from the American Academy of Nursing (AAN); and inaugural Fellow in the Academy of Diversity Leaders in Nursing. Dr. Malone was elected to two terms as president of the ANA, representing 180,000 nurses and served as the first African American general secretary of the United Kingdom Royal College of Nursing representing 400,000 nurses.

# About the Contributors

**Ann Bonner**, PhD, MA, BAppSc (Nurs), RN, MACN, MAICD, is head of the School of Nursing and Midwifery (Griffith University, Queensland, Australia), visiting research fellow, Kidney Health Service (Metro North Health Service, Queensland, Australia), Honorary Skou Professor, Aarhus University (Denmark), and adjunct professor (Queens University Belfast, UK). She is the deputy chair, Council of Deans of Nursing and Midwifery Australia and New Zealand. An experienced nurse leader with significant clinical, academic, and research experience across the health and higher education sectors for more than 30 years, Ann has attracted over $10 million in competitive research funding, has a distinguished record of publications (Scopus H-Index - 35, FWCI - 1.78), and has supervised doctoral students and nurse education at undergraduate and postgraduate levels. She is a member of ICN Education Expert Advisory Committee, a life-member of the Renal Society of Australasia, a member of the Australian Institute of Health and Welfare Chronic Kidney Disease Expert Advisory Group, and in 2021, was inducted into the International Nurse Researcher Hall of Fame.

**Janice Brewington**, PhD, RN, FADLN, FAAN, retired as chief program officer and director for the Center for Transformational Leadership at the NLN, where she implemented two year-long leadership programs: LEAD and the Leadership Development Program for Simulation Educators. She continues to manage these programs as an NLN consultant. She was assistant dean, interim dean, and provost and vice chancellor for academic affairs at North Carolina Agricultural and Technical (NC A&T) State University. Her educational background includes a BSN degree from NC A&T State University, an MSN degree from Emory University, and a PhD degree in health policy and administration from the School of Public Health, with a minor in organizational behavior from the School of Business, at the University of North Carolina at Chapel Hill. She also received a certificate from the Management and Leadership Institute at Harvard University. The American Academy of Nursing selected Dr. Brewington as a Living Legend. She is also a Fellow in the AAN, the A.K. Rice Institute for the Study of Social Systems, and the National Black Nurses Association's Academy of Diversity Leaders in Nursing. She has published articles and made presentations globally. Dr. Brewington has secured more than $30 million in grant funding.

**Kellie Bryant**, DNP, WHNP, CHSE, FSSH, FADLN, FAAN, serves as the director of the Center for Innovation in Education Excellence at the NLN. With more than 20 years of experience in nursing education and 15 years in simulation, she leads national efforts to advance teaching and learning through innovative strategies and technologies. In her role, Dr. Bryant oversees the development of faculty development programs and transformative educational tools that support nurse educators and improve learner outcomes. She plays a central role in the implementation of AI-driven software aimed at modernizing nursing education. Through strategic collaboration, she expands the NLN's innovation portfolio, aligning new technologies with the evolving needs of the nursing workforce. Dr. Bryant's work reflects a deep commitment to academic excellence, equitable education, and the integration of emerging technologies to prepare the next generation of nurses.

**Linda Christensen**, EdD, JD, RN, CNE, FAAN, is a nurse educator–administrator–lawyer. She has more than 35 years of experience in nursing education, ranging from teaching nursing assistant classes at a community college to teaching graduate nursing students. During her years as an education administrator, she served as program director (for various levels of nursing), dean of nursing, and vice president of academic affairs. As a lawyer, she has served as a civil litigator, in-house attorney, and legal writing instructor. For the past 30 years, Linda has served as an expert witness on various health- and education-related lawsuits. Linda has authored various chapters on legal issues in nursing education. She has served as a guest speaker on legal issues, with a particular focus on nursing education and the law. Linda is currently chief legal officer at the NLN.

**Nuhad Yazbik Dumit**, RN, MA, PhD, is a tenured professor and associate dean, coordinator of the PhD program and the chairperson of the Online Programs at the School of Nursing, American University of Beirut. She has several funded research projects, related publications, and invited presentations in international scientific conferences, focusing on nursing workforce issues. She served as a consultant locally and regionally to several higher education projects especially in the health disciplines, World Health Organization (WHO) Eastern Mediterranean Region Office and United Nations Population Fund Beirut on health projects. She served as the president of the Order of Nurses in Lebanon, June 2015–June 2018. In that capacity, she submitted several nursing regulation proposals for nursing education and practice and organized a regional symposium addressing the impact of refugee health care on the nursing workforce. She served as a member of the Scientific Steering Committee for the ICN Code of Ethics, currently serving as a member of the ICN Education Experts Advisory Committee. She received several honors and awards at the university, national, and international levels. She holds a BS in nursing and master's in education policy from the American University of Beirut, and a PhD in nursing from the University of Colorado, College of Nursing.

**Jan Jones-Schenk**, DHSc, RN, FAAN, FAADN, is executive dean emeritus of the Michael O. Leavitt School of Health at Western Governors University. The Leavitt School of Health is entirely competency-based, offering graduate and undergraduate degrees in nursing and the health professions. During her tenure, Dr. Jones-Schenk facilitated over 95,000 graduates and had strategic oversight for over 30,000 active students in all 50 states of the United States. She has served on multiple boards, including the ANA and American Nurses Credentialing Center where, as board chair, she implemented the first international Magnet research and implementation project. She is a Fellow of the Academy of Associate Degree Nursing and a Fellow of the AAN. Dr. Jones-Schenk has a master's degree in nursing administration and a doctorate in health sciences with an emphasis on global health. She has received the U.S. Distance Learning Association Award, Online Learning Consortium Digital Innovation Learning Award, and

Gates Foundation Prize. In 2022, she received the prestigious NLN Presidents' Award for innovation in nursing education. She is associate editor for the monthly leadership column for the *Journal of Continuing Education in Nursing*. Dr. Jones-Schenk is a national expert on competency-based education and learning science.

**Teddie Potter**, PhD, RN, FAAN, FNAP, is the director of the Center for Planetary Health and Environmental Justice at the School of Nursing at the University of Minnesota and a Fellow in the Institute on the Environment at the University. She is a board member of the Alliance of Nurses for Healthy Environments and the Planetary Health Report Card. She is a member of the AAN Environment and Public Health Expert Panel and the Steering Committee of the Planetary Health Alliance. She serves on the NAM's Action Collaborative on Decarbonizing the U.S. Health Sector; the Health and Medicine Division of the National Academy of Sciences, Engineering, and Medicine (NASEM); and the Climate Crossroads committee of NASEM. Her most recent work is with the ICN to promote Nursing for Planetary Health.

**Cynda Hylton Rushton**, PhD, RN, FAAN, is an international leader in bioethics and nursing, and is the Anne and George L. Bunting Professor of Clinical Ethics and Nursing at the Johns Hopkins Berman Institute of Bioethics and the School of Nursing. Dr. Rushton is the editor and author of *Moral Resilience: Transforming Moral Suffering in Healthcare* and co-creator of the Rushton Moral Resilience Scale. Dr. Rushton is the chief synergy strategist for Maryland's R3 Resilient Nurses Initiative, a statewide initiative to build resilience and ethical practice in nursing students, faculty and practicing nurses, and co-creator of the Mindful Ethical Practice and Resilience Academy.

**Patricia A. Sharpnack**, DNP, RN, CNE, NEA-BC, ANEF, FAAN, is past chair (2023–2025) of the NLN Board of Governors and current dean and Strawbridge Professor at Ursuline College, The Breen School of Nursing and Health Professions. She has held numerous leadership and board positions on regulatory bodies and served as the chief nursing officer for several health care agencies and as a leader in professional organizations at regional, national, and international levels. She was appointed to the Ohio Board of Nursing and was president for three terms, supervisory member, nursing education chair, and National Council of State Boards of Nursing delegate and committee member from 2014 through 2022. She is on the editorial board and reviewer for several refereed journals, has extensively published and presented at national and international conferences, and received numerous awards and recognition. She is a Fellow of both the NLN Academy of Nurse Educators and the AAN. Dr. Sharpnack received a diploma in nursing from St. Vincent Charity School of Nursing, a BSN from Ursuline College, an MSN from the University of Akron, a DNP from the Frances Payne Bolton School of Nursing at Case Western Reserve University, and a postgraduate certificate in health policy and media engagement from George Washington University.

**Teresa Shellenbarger**, DNP, RN, CNE, NEA-BC, ANEF, FAAN, is the executive director of the National League for Nursing Commission for Nursing Accreditation (NLN CNEA) where she oversees nursing accreditation activities for nursing programs across the education spectrum and around the globe. She is a distinguished university professor emeritus from Indiana University of Pennsylvania, where she served as the founding PhD program coordinator in the Department of Nursing and Allied Health Professions. She is a distinguished scholar and leader in nursing education and draws from her more than 30 years of teaching at the baccalaureate, master's, and doctoral levels to advance quality and excellence in nursing education. Dr. Shellenbarger is a respected expert and sought-after speaker on topics related to accreditation, program development and evaluation, innovative teaching strategies, clinical nursing education, faculty roles, and student issues in nursing education. She has an impressive record of national and international presentations and has published four books, numerous book chapters, and over 100 peer-reviewed journal articles. Dr. Shellenbarger is certified by the NLN as an academic nurse educator and an academic clinical nurse educator and was inducted as an inaugural Fellow in the NLN Academy of Nursing Education.

**Larry Simmons**, PhD, RN, CNE, NEA-BC, CGNC, FAAN, has been a nurse educator for 30 years and has worked as the director of the certified nurse educator program at the NLN for 12 years. He was responsible for the globalization of the nurse educator certifications, opening the program to nurse education faculty around the world. He has been responsible for the development of three new nurse educator certifications. He is a nationally and internationally known speaker on nursing education and nurse educator certification.

**Erna Snelgrove-Clarke**, PhD, RN, was most recently vice dean, Health Sciences, and director, School of Nursing, Queen's University (2019–2024). Currently, she holds the title as professor in the School of Nursing, Queen's University. She received her bachelor's degree in nursing from Memorial University of Newfoundland, her master's of nursing from Dalhousie University in Halifax, and her PhD (nursing) from McGill University in Montreal. Dr. Snelgrove-Clarke worked as a maternity nurse for 37 years. She has more than 32 years of research experience in various aspects of health care, focusing on women's health and knowledge translation. Professor Snelgrove-Clarke's program of research focuses on the identification of successful strategies for translating research evidence into maternal and women's health care. More specifically, this implementation involves changing provider behavior to use best evidence, thereby enhancing patient outcomes. She explores the transfer of knowledge through multiple methods, concentrating on the relationships of health care professionals, organizations, and decision makers. As a person-centered leader, she focuses on a healthful practice that is inclusive, collaborative, and respectful.

**Maxim Topaz**, PhD, RN, MA, FAAN, FIAHSI, FACMI, is an associate professor of nursing at Columbia University (NYC, USA). His research uses AI and innovative technologies to improve health care, including text/data mining and automated speech processing. He pioneered natural language processing for health care data and is currently focused on developing AI solutions for clinical decision-making. Dr. Topaz has published over 170 articles, and his research portfolio includes more than $20 million in federal and other funding. Dr. Topaz has experience in health policy, leadership, and entrepreneurship. He has clinical experience in internal and urgent medicine, a PhD from the University of Pennsylvania (USA), and a postdoctoral fellowship at Harvard Medical School (USA).

**Yolanda M. VanRiel**, PhD, RN, MEDSURG-BC, OCN, CNE, ACUE, ANEF, FAAN, is department chair of nursing at North Carolina Central University and brings 29 years of nursing experience, including 24 years in nursing education. She holds degrees from Richmond Community College, UNC Greensboro (BSN, MSN in Nursing Education), and UNC Chapel Hill (PhD in Nursing), along with certificates in Healthcare Disparities (UNC Chapel Hill) and Nursing Administration (Queens University of Charlotte). Dr. VanRiel is a Fellow in the NLN Academy of Nursing Education and AAN and holds certifications as a nurse educator, oncology nurse, and board-certified medical-surgical nurse. She actively contributes to professional organizations such as the ANA, Oncology Nursing Society, and Sigma Theta Tau. She currently serves as chair of the Board of Governors for the NLN (2025-2027) and is past president of the North Carolina League for Nursing. She previously served on the North Carolina Board of Nursing, including as vice chair (2018–2019). Dr. VanRiel has received numerous honors, including the NCNA Nurse Educator of the Year and the Great 100 Nurses of NC. Her research focuses on nursing education, health disparities, oncology, and provider–patient communication, and she has a strong record of scholarly presentations, publications, and grant work.

**Ilse Wallace**, PhD, RN, CNE, is a visionary nurse educator and executive leader with over 19 years of experience in fostering a dynamic and inclusive learning environment for a diverse student body. Ilse holds a bachelor's degree in Nursing and master's degree in Nursing Education from Florida Atlantic University and a PhD in Nursing from Barry University. Currently serving as the executive dean for Academic Quality at Chamberlain University, Ilse is dedicated to achieving superior academic outcomes and advancing the standards of nursing education. Ilse has proven leadership in curriculum and course development, assessment strategy, clinical learning experiences, and teaching and learning. Dr. Wallace is an alumnus of the NLN LEAD program, has published, co-authored an NLN vision statement on competency-based education, and presented at numerous conferences on nursing and higher education. Ilse is committed to driving excellence in nursing education and enhancing university programs through strategic initiatives and collaboration across programs, universities, and partners.

# Foreword

Strong nursing education today means strong health care tomorrow. Education is one of the critical pillars of the International Council of Nurses (ICN) because we know that investing in high-quality, competence-based education is key to producing the pipeline of well-prepared nursing graduates, advanced practice nurses, and nursing faculty that our world urgently needs. ICN's Education Experts Advisory Committee, with the invaluable support of the National League for Nursing (NLN), has been working diligently to address critical issues in nursing education worldwide. The Committee's work is part of ICN's legacy of deep commitment to nursing education, regulation, and professional and leadership development, including our new Leadership Center, which brings together all of ICN's leadership development programs.

The insights and recommendations that emerged from the NLN Utstein Global Conference for Expert Nurse Educators held in June 2025 represent a crucial contribution to our collective efforts to strengthen nursing education worldwide. This work is a significant step forward in addressing vital strategic issues and evidence-based solutions that will enrich and expand education at every level, from implementing unified standards for adequate practice hours and effective supervision to integrating hybrid and simulation-based learning with clinical mentorship, promoting the health and well-being of nurses and nurse educators, and ensuring competence and preparedness for digital transformations.

The urgency of advancing nursing education cannot be overstated. With a global shortage of 5.8 million nurses, every graduate matters. We are confronting enormous global health challenges ranging from the increasing health impacts of climate change and conflicts to aging populations, rising chronic diseases, and escalating mental health issues. Rapid advances in digital technology and artificial intelligence present many opportunities but also challenges in ensuring equity, educational competence, and faculty and graduate readiness. These issues are all compounded by current crises in health financing around the world, including substantial cuts in international development assistance and changes in funding availability that could limit access to nursing education and postgraduate programs. Strong nursing education that produces strong nursing workforces is vital to addressing all these current and future health care demands.

The 2025 World Health Organization State of the World's Nursing (SOWN) report, which ICN co-chaired, shows some progress with positive movement toward nursing as an all-graduate profession: approximately 84 percent of nurses globally are now prepared with a minimum of three to four years of education. However, we face major challenges. There are grave inequalities in both nursing education and workforce distribution around the world. For example, high-income countries have a tenfold higher density of nurses compared with low-income countries. While many countries have established high-level standards for education, we lack sufficient data about the quality of policies, enforcement mechanisms, and funding that support these standards. There also are significant variations in how closely education providers and regulatory bodies work together. The SOWN report also underscores the importance of seizing the opportunities of advanced practice nursing, which requires specialized education and is vital for making care accessible and strengthening primary health care, the key to Universal Health Coverage (UHC).

At this year's World Health Assembly, WHO member states unanimously voted to extend the Strategic Directions for Nursing and Midwifery to 2030 based on findings from the State of the World's Nursing report. The Strategic Directions include clear commitments to educating sufficient graduates at a practice-ready level to meet increasing demands on our health systems, to educating and enabling advanced practice nurses, and to ensuring that nursing education incorporates the most effective, up-to-date, and innovative learning designs.

We must continue to advocate to translate these commitments to real action to strengthen and adapt nursing education. That means calling for urgent investment in educating the practice-ready nurses of the future who can lead the transformation of care and in ensuring a sustainable pipeline of nursing faculty who are supported with fair working conditions. Nursing education is a fundamental building block of accessible, cost-effective care and achieving universal health coverage. It is a core component of reaching our global health goals and promoting health for all people. Let us work together to build educational systems and structures that empower and nurture the nursing profession to make quality care available to everyone.

*Pamela Cipriano, PhD, RN, NEA-BC, FAAN,*
*Immediate Past President, International Council of Nurses*
*Howard Catton, MA, BScEcon (Hons), RN,*
*Chief Executive Officer, International Council of Nurses*

# Quotation

Supporting the Utstein Project reflects a shared commitment to evidence-driven nursing leadership and safer patient care. Through the Health Carousel Foundation's partnership, we're proud to help advance research that strengthens clinical practice, improves outcomes, and elevates the nursing workforce for the communities we serve.

*– Health Carousel Foundation*

# Acknowledgments

The National League for Nursing is grateful for the generous sponsorship and co-sponsorship to host this first-ever nursing-focused Utstein meeting.

## Utstein Meeting Sponsors

Laerdal Foundation

Health Carousel

## Utstein Meeting Co-Sponsors

American Association of Colleges of Nursing

CHAMBERLAIN College of Nursing

GALEN COLLEGE OF NURSING®

nsna National Student Nurses' Association

NIGHTINGALE EDUCATION GROUP

The Editors also would like to thank the following persons (in alphabetical order) for their contributions to making the first ever nursing-focused Utstein meeting successful:

- Tigist Bishaw for coordinating communications with the nursing experts who attended the meeting and preparing name badges/meeting materials;
- Arielle Charles for coordinating flights for the nursing experts who attended the meeting;
- Taras Kalynych for coordinating flights for the nursing experts who attended the meeting;
- Debra Mayberry for coordinating lodging, catering, and onsite event logistics (and keeping us well-fed over the two days);
- Amy McGuire for managing the registration portal and assisting Tigist Bishaw with operational preparations; and
- India West for creating the onsite program for the nursing experts who attended the meeting.

# Table of Contents


*About the Authors* v

*About the Contributors* vii

*Foreword* xii

*Quotation* xiv

*Acknowledgments* xv

*List of Figures and Tables* xx

*List of Abbreviations* xxii

PART 1 **ISSUES FACING THE FUTURE OF NURSING EDUCATION 1**

CHAPTER 1 **Setting the Stage to Shape the Future of Nursing Education** 3
*Sandra Davis*

CHAPTER 2 **Implementing the Utstein Meeting Using a World Café Study Design** 8
*Gordon Lee Gillespie*

CHAPTER 3 **Focus Areas for the Future of Nursing Education** 23
*Gordon Lee Gillespie, Sandra Davis, Teresa Shellenbarger, Ilse Wallace, Janice Brewington, Patricia A. Sharpnack, Larry Simmons, Kellie Bryant, Linda Christensen, Yolanda M. VanRiel, and Beverly Malone*

PART 2 **COMPETENCY-BASED EDUCATION IN NURSING 31**

CHAPTER 4 **Overview of Competency-Based Education in Nursing** 33
*Jan Jones-Schenk*

CHAPTER 5 **Barriers and Strategies for Incorporating Competency-Based Education Into Nursing Education** 42
*Gordon Lee Gillespie and Sandra Davis*

PART 3 **ARTIFICIAL INTELLIGENCE 51**

CHAPTER 6 **Overview of Artificial Intelligence** 53
*Maxim Topaz*

CHAPTER 7 **Barriers and Strategies for Incorporating Artificial Intelligence Into Nursing Education** 67
*Gordon Lee Gillespie and Sandra Davis*

PART 4 **PLANETARY HEALTH 75**

CHAPTER 8 **Overview of Planetary Health** 77
*Teddie Potter*

CHAPTER 9 **Barriers and Strategies for Incorporating Planetary Health Constructs Into Nursing Education** 86
*Gordon Lee Gillespie and Sandra Davis*

PART 5 **NURSE AND NURSING FACULTY WELL-BEING 95**

CHAPTER 10 **Overview of Nurse and Nursing Faculty Well-Being** 97
*Cynda Hylton Rushton*

CHAPTER 11 **Barriers and Strategies for Incorporating Nurse and Nursing Faculty Well-Being Into Nursing Education** 109
*Gordon Lee Gillespie and Sandra Davis*

PART 6 **ADDRESSING THE GLOBAL NURSING FACULTY SHORTAGE 119**

CHAPTER 12 **Overview of the Global Nursing Faculty Shortage** 121
*Nuhad Yazbik Dumit, Patricia A. Sharpnack, Erna Snelgrove-Clarke, and Ann Bonner*

CHAPTER 13 **Barriers and Strategies for Addressing the Global Nursing Faculty Shortage** 132
*Gordon Lee Gillespie and Sandra Davis*

PART 7 **FINDING HOPE IN THE FUTURE** 143

CHAPTER 14 **Strategies and Confidence in the Future for Nursing Education at a Global Level** 145

*Gordon Lee Gillespie, Sandra Davis, Teresa Shellenbarger, Ilse Wallace, Janice Brewington, Patricia A. Sharpnack, Larry Simmons, Kellie Bryant, Linda Christensen, Yolanda M. VanRiel, and Beverly Malone*

*Appendix* 159

# List of Figures and Tables

LIST OF FIGURES

Figure 1.1 Application of Social Ecological Model to Priority Issues in Nursing Education 6

Figure 2.1 Example of Table Assignments by Session and Round 12

Figure 2.2 World Café Table Set With Basket of Supplies 13

Figure 2.3 World Café Room Is Set With Different-Colored Baskets to Facilitate Transitions Between Tables 13

Figure 2.4 Prelabeled Flip-Chart Pages 17

Figure 2.5 Group Photo of the Utstein Meeting Discussants, Table Hosts, and Support Team 20

Figure 4.1 CTUS Model for Competency-Based Nursing Education 37

Figure 8.1 The Evolution of the Planetary Boundaries Framework 78

Figure 8.2 Planetary Health: Protecting Human Health on a Rapidly Changing Planet 81

Figure 10.1 Social Ecological Framework 103

LIST OF TABLES

Table 2.1 Primary Professional Setting, World Health Organization Region, and Global Bank Income Level for the Countries in Which the World Café Discussants Worked (N=60) 11

Table 2.2 Questions Asked of Discussants by Session and Table 16

Table 2.3 Kappa Statistics for Each Round of Data Analysis 19

Table 8.1 Planetary Health Resources 83

Table 10.1 Selected Evidence-Informed Individual Interventions for Nurse and Nursing Faculty Well-Being 101

Table 10.2 Selected Evidence-Informed Systemic Interventions for Nurse and Nursing Faculty Well-Being 102

Table 14.1 Recommendations/Strategies for the Future of Nursing Education 153

# List of Abbreviations

| | |
|---|---|
| AACN | American Association of Colleges of Nursing |
| AI | Artificial Intelligence |
| ANA | American Nurses Association |
| AONL | American Organization of Nurse Leaders |
| AR | Augmented Reality |
| CBE | Competency-Based Education |
| GPA | Grade Point Average |
| H&P | History and Physical |
| ICN | International Council of Nurses |
| LGBTQ | Lesbian, Gay, Bisexual, Transgender, Queer |
| NASEM | National Academies of Sciences, Engineering, and Medicine |
| NCSBN | National Council of State Boards of Nursing |
| NLN | National League for Nursing |
| STEM | Science, Technology, Engineering, and Mathematics |
| U.S. | United States |
| VR | Virtual Reality |
| WHO | World Health Organization |

PART 1

# Issues Facing the Future of Nursing Education

1

# Setting the Stage to Shape the Future of Nursing Education

**Sandra Davis**

## INTRODUCTION

Globally, nurses are vital to every sector of society. Representing the largest segment of the global health care workforce, nurses provide over 80 percent of direct patient care (Nemati-Vakilabad et al., 2025; World Health Organization [WHO], 2025). Although the indispensable role of nurses in health care facilities is well recognized, their power and expertise extend beyond traditional health care settings (Whelan, n.d.). Working in industry, schools and universities, nonprofit organizations, government, and independent entrepreneurship roles, nurses are integral to shaping solutions and tackling the most pressing global challenges.

Nursing education is central to nurses' ability to lead across contexts in a complex and rapidly changing world. As the world evolves, so must nursing education. Nursing education is fundamental to safety, high-quality, and equitable health and social care. However, there is growing concern that nursing education has not kept pace with advances in knowledge and technology and the overall accelerating rate of transformation in a volatile world. Major reports over the past two decades have consistently championed the need to revolutionize nursing education. The Carnegie Study of 2009 called for a *radical* transformation in nursing education (Benner et al., 2009). The State of the World's Nursing 2020 report urged substantial investment to significantly expand nursing education, inclusive of faculty, students, and infrastructure (WHO, 2020). The 2021 Future of Nursing Report 2020–2030 called for a *rapid* transformation in nursing education (National Academies of Sciences, Engineering, and Medicine [NASEM], 2021).

Nursing education is at a critical juncture (National Council of State Boards of Nursing [NCSBN], 2023). Nurses must be ready to practice in an era of flux amidst geopolitical instability, conflict, migration, climate impacts, emerging infectious diseases, transformation driven by artificial intelligence (AI), workforce shortages, and health and social inequities. Nursing programs must balance meeting these demands with faculty shortages, burnout, constrained budgets, entrenched systems and structures, traditional curricula, and long-standing modes of delivery, assessment, and evaluation.

## BACKGROUND

The origins of nursing education date back two centuries. Over a span of 227 years, nursing education transformed from physician-taught apprenticeships to academically rigorous university programs taught by nurses (Whelan, n.d.). Blood pressure measurement, a standard skill for nurses, was once considered a diagnostic procedure performed only by physicians. Today, nurses are educated and trained by nurse educators to intubate and perform other advanced skills, including managing sedation during surgical procedures, making clinical diagnoses, and prescribing medications. However, poised at a crossroads, the question is: What will the future bring for nursing education?

The National League for Nursing (NLN, 2025b) Research Priorities in Nursing Education 2024–2027 identify critical gaps and emerging trends in nursing education and provide a roadmap to guide nurse educators as they prepare for the future. The explosive growth of AI will undoubtedly transform how nurse educators teach and how students learn. In addition, competency-based education (CBE) is being examined more closely as a model for the future of nursing education. Research in nursing education will be essential for closing significant gaps that currently exist in understanding how to effectively integrate AI and CBE into nursing education. Alongside AI and CBE, planetary health, well-being, and faculty workforce shortages remain key priorities for advancing nursing education into the future (International Council of Nurses [ICN], 2023; ICN, 2024; NASEM, 2021; NCSBN, 2025). Nursing education researchers who generate knowledge and translate evidence into new and innovative teaching and learning strategies will be vital to addressing gaps in knowledge, assessment, and evaluation. However, first, a global effort is needed to convene and build consensus on priority topics in nursing education, as well as on the strategies, facilitators, and barriers to transforming nursing education for the future. This information is essential to inform current decisions on critical nursing education issues that will influence the profession for years. The stakes are high given the urgent need for nurse educators to prepare students for the realities of practice in an increasingly complex, rapidly evolving world.

## SIGNIFICANCE

Now more than ever, intensifying world challenges demand a practice-ready global nursing workforce. Worldwide, there is an urgent need to transform nursing education to prepare nurses who can: (1) *adapt* to rapidly evolving health care needs and the exponential growth of AI; (2) *respond* to workforce shortages, climate impacts, migration, conflicts, and disasters; and (3) *lead* in developing innovative solutions that support well-being and address systemic barriers to advancing health equity.

There are thousands of nursing education institutions around the world. As expected, these institutions vary in program levels and time to degree completion; educational systems, classification standards, and accreditation requirements; local and cultural contexts; and available resources. Albeit needed, attaining meaningful collaboration and achieving consensus on co-creating a practice-ready global workforce is an extraordinarily daunting and, some may even say, unattainable goal. However, grounded in its mission to promote "excellence in nursing education to build a strong and diverse nursing workforce to advance the health of our nation and the global community," the NLN (2025a) recognized that the time to act is now.

## PURPOSE

On June 7–8, 2025, the NLN hosted the landmark NLN Utstein Conference on the Future of Nursing Education in Helsinki, Finland. The purpose of this meeting was to assemble global thought leaders in nursing education, clinical practice, and regulation to help determine a global vision for the future of nursing education. Sixty leaders from 13 countries, representing all six WHO regions, participated in this event. The specific aims for this meeting were to (1) identify priorities for the future of nursing education and (2) describe strategies, facilitators, and barriers for selected nursing education topics.

## THEORETICAL FRAMEWORK

The issues impacting the future of nursing education are complex, interrelated, and intersecting. Moreover, these issues influence and are influenced by multiple systems and factors within those systems, creating a dynamic reciprocity that underscores the need for a unifying and comprehensive framework (Clark et al., 2024). Each educational priority and its associated strategies, facilitators, and barriers exist within an interdependent system that is impacted by (1) nurse educators/faculty; (2) nursing programs and the schools, colleges, and/or universities that nursing programs may be situated within; (3) national, societal, and nursing norms, laws, and policies; and (4) the international nursing community. The path forward for transforming nursing education is dynamic, reciprocal, and interdependent, requiring collaboration and communication among global thought leaders in nursing education, clinical practice, and regulation to co-create a shared global vision for the future of nursing education.

To inform the collaboration, communication, and outcomes of the NLN Utstein Conference on the Future of Nursing Education, a theoretical framework was adopted that emphasizes the integration of systems thinking within and across multiple levels. The social ecological model (Bronfenbrenner, 1977) provides a comprehensive systems framework for examining complex issues that demand a holistic perspective (Dahlberg & Krug, 2006; Gillespie et al., 2025). Moreover, this model allows for comparing and contrasting both the unique characteristics and the interconnectedness of global nursing education challenges. The framework for this Utstein meeting and associated research is presented in four levels based on the social ecological model: (1) faculty/nurse educator (microsystem); (2) program, school, college, and university (mesosystem); (3) national (exosystem); and (4) international/global (macrosystem).

The faculty/nurse educator level focuses on all factors related to nursing faculty/nurse educators (see Figure 1.1). The program, school, college, and university level includes all factors related to a nursing program and any associated school, college, and/or university and its broader academic setting, including other interprofessional disciplines and the external/local community. The national level includes national/societal and nursing norms, associations, policies, laws, and regulations, as well as issues affecting nursing education, clinical practice, health, and health care. Finally, the international level focuses on international/nursing and global associations and policies, as well as issues affecting nursing education, clinical practice, health, and health care.

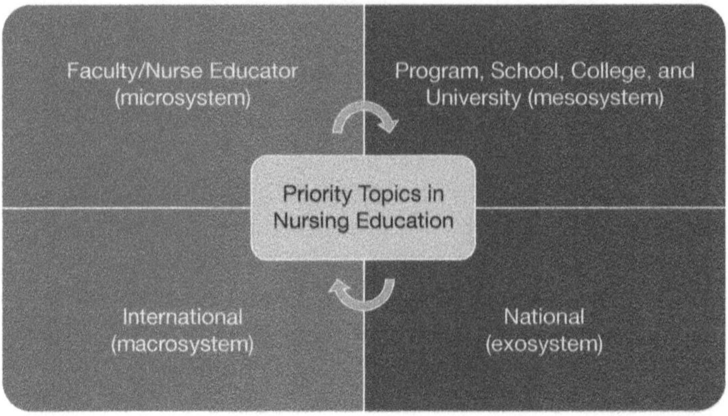


**FIGURE 1.1:** Application of Social Ecological Model to Priority Issues in Nursing Education

## BOOK STRUCTURE

This book is a comprehensive guide to the first of its kind global Utstein meeting to develop a vision for the future of nursing education using a World Café approach. The extraordinary two-day journey consisted of four short presentations, one panel discussion, and six iterative working sessions, generating 3,296 data points in total. The resulting analysis and summary of these findings are featured in this book. The book is designed to be read either in its entirety for a comprehensive understanding or consulted selectively, as each chapter serves as a self-contained resource.

Chapter 2 details the methods and implementation of the Utstein meeting, describing how using a World Café project design ensured that every participant's perspective contributed to robust findings that created a vision for nursing education by 2030 and beyond. Chapter 3 reports the future educational priorities, strategies, and innovations recommended by Utstein meeting participants as necessary for nursing education and clinical practice.

Chapters 4, 6, 8, 10, and 12 describe the current state of nursing education across five priority topics. Although the original presentations and panel only provided an overview to orient participants to a given topic, the chapters in this book offer much greater detail, providing context and description for readers.

Chapters 5, 7, 9, 11, and 13 report the findings of the data analysis, detailing priorities in nursing education and the strategies, facilitators, and barriers for the five selected priority nursing education topics. These findings from the transformative meeting will serve as a foundation for galvanizing leadership among nurse educators, holding systems and structures accountable for change and grounding educational innovation in research evidence, while setting the stage for global collaboration and co-creation to equip a practice-ready workforce. Chapter 14 provides a synthesis of the discussion and implications derived from the Utstein meeting. Implications are presented at the microsystem, mesosystem, exosystem, and macrosystem levels based on Bronfenbrenner's (1977) social ecological model.

# CONCLUSION

The NLN Utstein Conference on the Future of Nursing Education marks a pivotal moment in shaping the future of nursing on an international scale. By bringing together leaders and experts from diverse backgrounds (e.g., academia, clinical practice, regulation, gender, race), countries, and WHO regions, the meeting fostered collaborative dialogue and generated consensus, insights, and actionable outcomes on the most pressing issues in nursing education. This book can serve as the catalyst to fuel the transformation of nursing education and influence clinical practice and regulation.

## *References*


Benner, P., Sutphen, M., Leonard, V., & Day, L. (2009). *Educating nurses: A call for radical transformation*. Jossey-Bass.

Bronfenbrenner, U. (1977). Toward an experimental ecology of human development. *American Psychologist, 32*(7), 513–531. https://doi.org/10.1037/0003-066X.32.7.513

Clark, C., Davis, S., Kuhl, L., Priddy, K. D., & Robinson, M. D. (2024). Conceptualizing the influence of diversity, equity, inclusion, and belonging on professional identity in nursing. *The Journal of Continuing Education in Nursing, 55*(10), 493–499. https://doi.org/10.3928/00220124-20240909-01

Dahlberg, L. L., & Krug, E. G. (2006). Violence a global public health problem. *Ciência & Saúde Coletiva, 11*(2), 277–292. https://doi.org/10.1590/S1413-81232006000200007

Gillespie, G. L., Meyer, H. A., Bakas, T., & Smith, C. R. (2025). A content analysis defining research-focused faculty success. *Nursing Outlook, 73*(1), 102312. https://doi.org/10.1016/j.outlook.2024.102312

International Council of Nurses. (2023). *Position statement: Digital health transformation and nursing practice*. International Council of Nurses. https://www.icn.ch/sites/default/files/2023-08/ICN%20Position%20Statement%20Digital%20Health%20FINAL%2030.06_EN.pdf

International Council of Nurses. (2024). *Position statement: Nurses, climate change and health*. International Council of Nurses. https://www.icn.ch/sites/default/files/2024-11/Nurses%20climate%20change%20health%20PS_EN.pdf

National Academies of Sciences, Engineering, and Medicine. (2021). *The future of nursing 2020–2030: Charting a path to achieve health equity.* The National Academies Press. https://doi.org/10.17226/25982

National Council of State Boards of Nursing. (2023). The NCSBN 2023 environmental scan: Nursing at a crossroads—An opportunity for action. *Journal of Nursing Regulation, 13*(4), supplement S1–S48. https://doi.org/10.1016/S2155-8256(23)00006-6

National Council of State Boards of Nursing. (2025). The 2025 NCSBN environmental scan: Going beyond. *Journal of Nursing Regulation, 15*(4), S1–S48. https://www.journalofnursingregulation.com/article/S2155-8256(25)00038-9/fulltext

National League for Nursing. (2025a). *Mission and strategic plan*. National League for Nursing. https://www.nln.org/about/about/mission-and-strategic-plan

National League for Nursing. (2025b). *NLN research priorities in nursing education 2024-2027*. National League for Nursing. https://www.nln.org/education/grants-scholarships/research-priorities-in-nursing-education

Nemati-Vakilabad, R., Kamalifar E., Jamshidinia M., & Mirzaei, A. (2025). Assessing the relationship between nursing process competency and work environment among clinical nurses: A cross-sectional correlational study. *BMC Nursing*, *24*, 134. https://doi.org/10.1186/s12912-025-02760-3

Whelan, J. C. (n.d.). *American nursing: An introduction to the past*. Penn Nursing. https://www.nursing.upenn.edu/nhhc/american-nursing-an-introduction-to-the-past/

World Health Organization. (2020). *State of the world's nursing 2020: Investing in education, jobs and leadership*. World

Health Organization. https://www.who.int/publications/i/item/9789240003279
World Health Organization. (2025, May 12). *Nursing workforce grows, but inequities threaten global health goals*. World Health Organization. https://www.who.int/news/item/12-05-2025-nursing-workforce-grows-but-inequities-threaten-global-health-goals

# 2

# Implementing the Utstein Meeting Using a World Café Study Design

**Gordon Lee Gillespie**

## UTSTEIN STYLE MEETING

The Utstein (pronounced as ut-STINE) style meeting is a specific style of meeting that originated in 1990 at the Utstein Abbey in Stavanger, Norway, and initially focused on uniform reporting of out-of-hospital cardiac arrest data (Otto et al., 2021). Since 1990, additional Utstein style meetings have focused on a wide range of topics, including cardiac arrest, trauma, prehospital and disaster care, veterinary cardiac arrest, newborn and maternal survival, and stroke. Two additional meetings focused specifically on education in resuscitation and on setting a research agenda for simulation-based health care education. Prior to our Utstein meeting, only two meetings were held outside of the Utstein Abbey, and no meetings ever focused on nursing. Our meeting was the first focused on nursing and nursing education.

The typical Utstein style meeting begins with a cohort of international experts separating into smaller groups. The experts then rotate among tables to discuss various topics and refine proposed solutions (Rudd et al., 2020). At the end of the discussion sessions, the meeting chairs present the results and facilitate debate among the experts. After the meeting, the chairs host teleconferences to finalize their Utstein meeting recommendations. Ultimately, the final report is approved through consensus of the cohort of international experts. For our meeting, we used an adapted Utstein style based on a

World Café study design, which is a qualitative and participatory method (Albrecht et al., 2022; Maloney & Harper, 2021; Masse-Grenier et al., 2024; McConnell et al., 2024; Schiele et al., 2022).

## STUDY DESIGN

The World Café, which originated in 1995 (Brown et al., 2005), is similar to focus groups; however, the method differs in that multiple, different but related, discussions occur simultaneously (Mamo et al., 2024; Schiele et al., 2022). The World Café method also allows for far more discussants than is feasible with a traditional focus group method (Albrecht et al., 2022; Schiele et al., 2022). A critical aspect of the World Café method is its ability to foster diverse perspectives, promote inclusion of all discussants, support collective discussion, and produce actionable knowledge (Albrecht et al., 2022; Brown et al., 2005; Masse-Grenier et al., 2024; McConnell et al., 2024; Schiele et al., 2022; Zadvinskis et al., 2025). Ultimately, this method can yield "a greater wisdom that is found only in the collective" (Brown et al., 2005, p. xv).

Similar to an Utstein style meeting, the World Café method begins with a session overview of a topic followed by discussants exploring a question at a café-style table. After a given period of time, discussants randomly move to a different table for another round of discussion. During the second and subsequent rounds, discussions focus on the same question (Mamo et al., 2024; Schiele et al., 2022); however, different tables may discuss different "standing" questions, or all tables may address the same question. At the end of the session of multiple discussion rounds, discussants reconvene for a large-group debriefing known as the harvest. The duration for each round varies (e.g., 10–40 minutes; Albrecht et al., 2022; Azulai et al., 2022; McConnell et al., 2024; Schiele et al., 2022; Zadvinskis et al., 2025), and a World Café itself could span just a few hours to several days, be a standalone event, or be attached to the end of a national symposium as a special session (Azulai et al., 2022; Zadvinskis et al., 2025).

### Advantages and Limitations

As a qualitative and participatory method, the World Café has many advantages. The key advantage is its ability to solicit "rich data from a varied group of stakeholders" (Mamo et al., 2024, p. 4). The continuous rounds of discussion promote an iterative and evolving outcome, help keep the conversations focused, and promote creativity of ideas (Maloney & Harper, 2021; Masse-Grenier et al., 2024; Schiele et al., 2022). As discussants work through the iterative process, they have the opportunity to revisit, review, and challenge information from prior rounds (Mamo et al., 2024). The final product is based on collaborative intelligence rather than the perspective of a single or few strong personalities who could have dominated a discussion (Ghafili et al., 2023).

Despite these strengths, the World Café method has two key limitations. First, dominant personalities still can affect the ability of other discussants to voice their opinions during a round (Azulai et al., 2022). However, the World Café's small group format and random reassignment to subsequent tables lessen the intimidation experienced in large groups and remove the power imbalance that could occur in the same group throughout the event (Ghafili et al., 2023). This structure allows every voice to carry equal weight and make a meaningful contribution to each conversation (Azulai et al., 2022). Second, the format limits the ability to probe for deeper context and meaning due to the shortened time frames of each round and not knowing which individual provided what information (Maloney & Harper, 2021). The final information is based on the collective and not an individual. However, discussants are given an opportunity during a harvest session to add any missed context or meaning.

## SETTING, SAMPLE, AND RECRUITMENT

Using a World Café method, the Utstein meeting took place in Helsinki, Finland, on June 7–8, 2025. This location was chosen because Helsinki was the site of the International Council of Nurses' (ICN) biannual Congress. By scheduling the World Café adjacent to this international event, discussants were able to reduce travel expenses and also the number of days they needed to be away from their normal responsibilities.

The World Café method enabled international experts to join and discuss a chosen topic (McConnell et al., 2024), specifically the future of nursing education. A purposive sample of experts was selected for inclusion (Masse-Grenier et al., 2024; McConnell et al., 2024). Experts were selected based on their national/international recognition as scholars in nursing education (e.g., member of the ICN Education Experts Advisory Committee, past national nursing organization leader). The Appendix lists the international experts who participated in the Utstein meeting. Recruitment efforts emphasized representation of six World Health Organization (WHO) regions as well as the Global World Bank's (2025) country income levels. Table 2.1 lists the countries where the discussants worked. Two experts from Africa were ultimately unable to attend due to difficulties obtaining visas to travel to Finland.

Initial solicitation emails were sent in February 2025, followed by reminder emails. In addition, the project team (Gordon Gillespie, Sandra Davis, and Beverly Malone) personally contacted potential discussants to notify them of the invitation and how to RSVP. The solicitation emails included a link for participants to respond "Yes" or "No" to attendance, as well as to provide details on their emergency contact information and any accessibility or accommodation needs during the event or related to the venue.

## ROLES OF WORLD CAFÉ ATTENDEES

There are three roles associated with the World Café meeting, World Café leaders, table hosts, and discussants. World Café leaders planned and oversaw all aspects of the Utstein meeting. Table hosts served as moderators for discussions with persons at their table and were selected based on their content expertise on the overall focus of the World Café topics, allowing for ongoing discussion and deeper exploration (Mamo et al., 2024). The Appendix provides a list of the table hosts. Lastly, discussants served as participants during the Utstein meeting.

### World Café Leaders

Gillespie and Davis served as World Café leaders. They started the Utstein meeting with a description of the World Café procedures (Mamo et al., 2024; Schiele et al., 2022). They did

**TABLE 2.1**

**Primary Professional Setting, World Health Organization Region, and Global Bank Income Level for the Countries in Which the World Café Discussants Worked (N=60)**

| Demographic characteristic | n | % |
|---|---|---|
| Primary professional setting | | |
| Academia | 38 | 63.3 |
| Health care organization/clinical practice | 3 | 5.0 |
| Professional society/association | 13 | 21.7 |
| Federal agency | 1 | 1.7 |
| Private industry | 5 | 8.3 |
| World Health Organization region | | |
| Africa | 1 | 1.7 |
| Americas | 47 | 78.3 |
| Eastern Mediterranean | 4 | 6.7 |
| Europe | 3 | 5.0 |
| South-East Asia | 3 | 5.0 |
| Western Pacific | 2 | 3.3 |
| Global Bank income level | | |
| High income | 51 | 85.0 |
| Upper middle income | 3 | 5.0 |
| Lower middle income | 6 | 10.0 |
| Low income | 0 | 0.0 |

not participate in conversations or serve as table hosts (Albrecht et al., 2022; Azulai et al., 2022). However, they did mingle and listen to rounds of discussion without disturbing the process (Albrecht et al., 2022; Azulai et al., 2022).

## Table Hosts

During each round of discussion, table hosts (moderators) followed a set procedure using detailed directions or guidance at their tables (Mamo et al., 2024; Schiele et al., 2022). Table hosts were identifiable by their name tags (Albrecht et al., 2022). Although table hosts participate in discussions at some World Cafés (Albrecht et al., 2022; Zadvinskis et al., 2025), in our World Café, table hosts waited until everyone at their table contributed before they spoke to prevent a stifling of the conversation and idea generation. Table hosts generated notes based on each discussion (Mamo et al., 2024; Masse-Grenier et al., 2024; Schiele et al., 2022) and helped keep the discussions focused without affirming or contradicting what was discussed (Mamo et al., 2024), allowing them to remain impartial and not influence the discussion. Table hosts remained at the same table for each round asking the same question to new discussants (Mamo et al., 2024; Schiele et al., 2022; Zadvinskis et al., 2025). As new discussants arrived at their table for the new round, table hosts summarized key points (Albrecht et al., 2022; Ghafili et al., 2023; Masse-Grenier et al., 2024; Maloney & Harper, 2021; McConnell et al., 2024; Schiele et al., 2022).

# PROCEDURES

## Training

Prior to the World Café, table hosts (moderators) received a guidebook detailing the procedures they would facilitate. They also received training about managing the table discussions (Mamo et al., 2024; Masse-Grenier et al., 2024; Schiele et al., 2022). During and after the training, they were given time to practice asking the questions (Zadvinskis et al., 2025).

## Preparation

The World Café environment needs to promote a hospitable, café-like environment (Brown et al., 2005). As they arrived, discussants were greeted as though arriving at an actual café by World Café leaders and Utstein meeting support staff (Brown et al., 2005). Discussants were shown to the registration desk, where support staff provided general information about the multiple purposes of their name badge—it listed the order of their table assignments (see Figure 2.1), which will be described later. Table hosts also warmly greeted discussants as they arrived at their initial table.

To further provide a café experience, the tables were set with NLN-colored baskets atop white linen (see Figure 2.2). These baskets also served as storage for the World Café supplies (i.e., ink pens, markers, sticky notes). The color of the baskets provided a visual indicator for the cluster of tables: dark blue for tables 1–3; teal for tables 4–6; and gold for tables 7–9 (see Figure 2.3). Flowers or other adornments were not used in an effort to reduce costs and prevent allergen exposures. In addition, we limited the number of chairs at each table to seven to promote comfort and to allow discussants to spread out their sticky notes as they were generated, which also limited the number of discussants invited to this inaugural meeting.

Before starting the Utstein meeting, discussants received welcome remarks from key representatives. First, Beverly Malone, president and chief executive officer for the National League for Nursing (NLN), welcomed the audience. Second, Andrew Lingo,

| | a | b | c |
|---|---|---|---|
| **Priorities** | 3 | 5 | 7 |
| **CBE** | 2 | 8 | 5 |
| **AI** | 7 | 5 | 2 |
| **Planet** | 2 | 8 | 6 |
| **Well-Being** | 3 | 7 | 5 |
| **Faculty** | 6 | 2 | 9 |

**FIGURE 2.1:** Example of Table Assignments by Session and Round

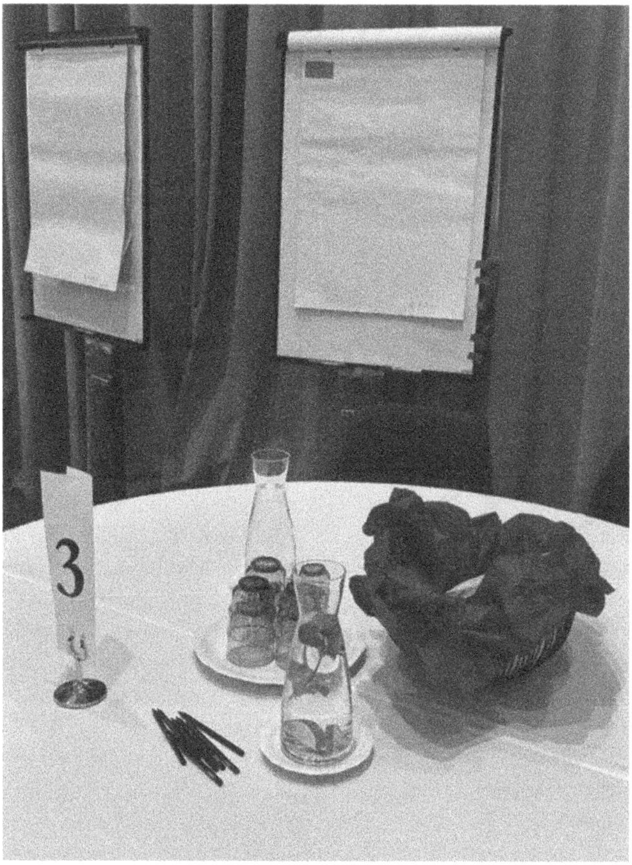


FIGURE 2.2: World Café Table Set With Basket of Supplies

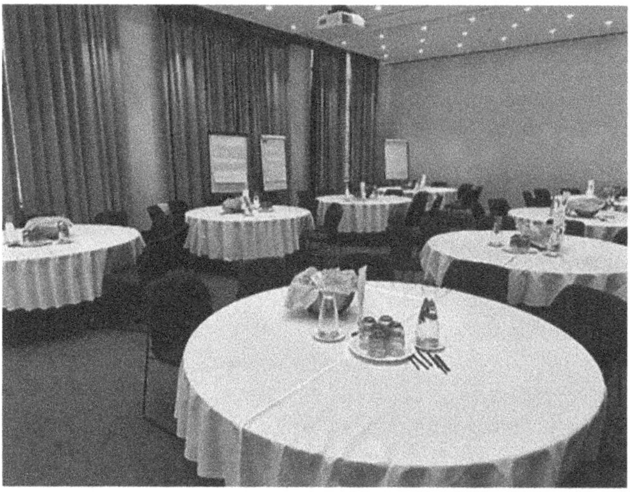

FIGURE 2.3: World Café Room Is Set With Different-Colored Baskets to Facilitate Transitions Between Tables

executive director for Health Carousel Foundation, and Earl Dalton, chief clinical officer and vice president clinical services, provided greetings. Third, a prerecorded message was delivered by Howard Catton, chief executive officer of the ICN. Fourth, a prerecorded message was delivered by Pamela Cipriano, president at that time of the ICN. Fifth, Amy Kline provided greetings on behalf of the Laerdal Foundation.

## World Café Session 1

In order to ensure focused sessions, a trial session took place (Albrecht et al., 2022). This initial (and trial) session focused on generating ideas and practicing the method. Discussants were randomly assigned to their initial table, and each World Café table responded to the single question:

- What are the educational priorities, strategies, and innovations needed for nursing education and clinical practice by 2030 and beyond?

Although there is no limit to the number of discussion rounds in a single session, we limited our number of discussion rounds to three per session. Round 1 lasted approximately 20 minutes. At the start of the round, the table host read the question aloud, and a printed copy of the question was placed on each table. Discussants were encouraged to document their thoughts or ideas on sticky notes (Azulai et al., 2022; Gillespie et al., 2025; Masse-Grenier et al., 2024), using provided ink pens and markers (Zadvinskis et al., 2025). There was no limit to the number of recommendations per round or session (Mamo et al., 2024). Table hosts also invited discussants to talk or describe what they had written on their sticky notes, although this was not required (Zadvinskis et al., 2025). Table hosts attached the sticky notes to flip-chart pages, and as the pages filled, they removed them from the easel and attached them to the wall next to the table. Near the end of the discussion round, the table host provided a summary of the discussion, allowing discussants to correct or add context. Table hosts then affixed any remaining sticky notes to the flip chart for future rounds of discussants to see them (Azulai et al., 2022). Discussants then moved to the next table (Brown et al., 2005), which was randomly preassigned, and the process was repeated.

Round 2 lasted approximately 20 minutes. During this round, table hosts read the question and provided a synopsis of the Round 1 discussion. Discussants could propose new recommendations or remove old ones if perceived as unrealistic (Mamo et al., 2024). The table hosts reported that no recommendations were removed during this round (or any future session or round). At the end of Round 2, table hosts provided a summary again. Discussants then moved to the next randomly assigned table, and Round 3 began.

Round 3 lasted approximately 15 minutes. Discussants remained at their table after idea generation had ended and the table hosts had provided the concluding summary. Discussants had five minutes to vote for what they perceived as the most important priorities, strategies, and/or innovations noted at their current table from all three rounds of discussion. Colored sticker dots were used for voting (Gillespie et al., 2025; Mamo et al., 2024; McConnell et al., 2024; Schiele et al., 2022). Each participant was given five colored dots. They were permitted to apply more than one dot to a particular priority, strategy, or innovation across a minimum of two priorities, strategies, and/or innovations. This voting process allowed discussants to see key results and to draw conclusions, rather than focusing on case exceptions or a particular point that one participant was passionate about (Schiele et al., 2022). The session concluded at the end of the voting, and discussants left the room for their break. The World Café leaders took pictures of the flip-chart pages and collected the sticky note data (Albrecht et al., 2022; Azulai et al., 2022; Gillespie et al., 2025). The data were secured in a different room for later analysis. The conference room was then prepared for the next World Café session.

## World Café Sessions 2–6

Brown et al. (2005) and McConnell et al. (2024) suggested that a plenary session before the World Café conversation rounds could help stimulate and focus the discussions (McConnell et al., 2024). In the remaining World Café sessions, we started with a 20-minute presentation (Sessions 2–5) or panel session followed by a 10-minute question-and-answer period (Session 6). These plenary sessions provided context about specific topics: CBE (Session 2), AI (Session 3), planetary health (Session 4), nurse and nursing faculty well-being (Session 5), and developing nurses to be faculty (Session 6). The World Café rounds commenced after each plenary session. Each session had three rounds and followed a similar format to that of Session 1, which focused on the overall future of nursing education. The questions for tables during Sessions 2–6 varied by table cluster. Ghafili et al. (2023) recommended that questions focus on the obstacles (barriers), solutions, and courses of action for each topic. In addition, the questions asked needed to matter to discussants (Brown et al., 2005). Table 2.2 highlights the session questions by table, respectively.

Procedures for changing tables after Rounds 1 and 2 as well as voting during Round 3 modeled those of Session 1. Similarly, World Café leaders took pictures of the flip charts and collected all of the data at the end of each session (Albrecht et al., 2022; Azulai et al., 2022; Gillespie et al., 2025).

## Harvest Sessions

After the focused sessions, World Café leaders led a series of "harvest sessions," which are similar to debriefing sessions but focused on the overall ideas generated and not the process itself (Maloney & Harper, 2021). These sessions increased data trustworthiness by allowing discussants to state any missing thoughts or ideas (Maloney & Harper, 2021). The harvest process started with World Café leaders reading the discussion questions for Session 2 and providing an overview of the findings based on the highest number of votes, followed by the table hosts and discussants providing additional responses, clarifications, and context. This process was repeated for Sessions 3–6.

During the final harvest session, the leading priorities, strategies, and innovations from Session 1 were addressed. They were clustered by an investigator-developed theme, and each World Café table focused on harvesting the items for that theme. The theme clusters were based on a preliminary review of the data and were not used for the analysis reported later in Chapter 3. Zadvinskis et al. (2025) described a fluid session where discussants came and went on their own schedule and visited as many tables as they wanted. Consistent with this approach, discussants were encouraged to move about the room visiting as many or as few tables as they wanted. At each table, the table hosts encouraged further dialogue and allowed discussants to vote on the priorities,

**TABLE 2.2**

**Questions Asked of Discussants by Session and Table**

| Session | Questions |
|---|---|
| Session 2 – CBE in Nursing | ➤ What are the barriers and strategies to overcome those barriers to implement CBE globally by 2030? [tables 1–3]<br>➤ What resources and assessment tools are needed for implementation of CBE? [tables 4–6]<br>➤ What are the minimum competencies needed for CBE in nursing? [tables 7–9] |
| Session 3 – AI | ➤ What are the strategies to promote the use of AI in nursing education and clinical practice? [tables 1–3]<br>➤ What strategies are needed to generate and translate innovative AI teaching and learning practice? [tables 4–6]<br>➤ What are the challenges and barriers to maintaining faculty competence on the rapid evolution of AI? [tables 7–9] |
| Session 4 – Planetary Health | ➤ What are the barriers and proposed solutions for the integration of planetary health into nursing curricula? [tables 1–3]<br>➤ What strategies can be used by faculty to prepare students to contribute to planetary health research, policy, and advocacy? [tables 4–6]<br>➤ What is the impact of planetary health to nursing education? [tables 7–9] |
| Session 5 – Nurse and Nursing Faculty Well-Being | ➤ What is nurse well-being? [tables 1–3]<br>➤ What are the barriers to nurse well-being? [tables 4–6]<br>➤ What are proposed solutions to creating sustainable healthy work environments where students, nurses, and nurse educators can thrive? [tables 7–9] |
| Session 6 – Addressing the Global Nursing Faculty Shortage | ➤ What are the barriers and proposed solutions for recruiting and retaining nursing faculty in your country? [tables 1–3]<br>➤ What strategies can be used to create nurse educator pathways in your country? [tables 4–6]<br>➤ What strategies can be used to promote diversity of the faculty in your country? [tables 7–9] |

strategies, and/or innovations they deemed most important for the future of nursing education (Mamo et al., 2024). Discussants were given two colored dots at each table to select where future resources should be prioritized for the future of nursing education on a global level (Mamo et al., 2024). In addition, sticky notes and space on the flip-chart page were provided for discussants to document their thoughts for the context of their voting. At the end, table hosts also voted at each table.

## HUMAN SUBJECTS PROTECTIONS

The research conducted during the Utstein meeting was approved by the University of Cincinnati Institutional Review Board (IRB # 2025-0250). At registration, each discussant was given a letter of information for research and also an overview of the research.

Their rights as human subjects also were presented to the discussants. As the principal investigator for the research, Gillespie also was available to answer any questions. Throughout the meeting, we reminded discussants not to put their name on any sticky note to maintain the confidentiality of their data.

Consistent with the World Café method, no identifiable demographic data were collected from discussants (Azulai et al., 2022). In addition, discussion rounds were not audio recorded (Azulai et al., 2022), and only publicly available demographic data, such as their WHO region, country, country's income level, and occupation/role, were collected.

## DATA MANAGEMENT, ANALYSIS, AND TRUSTWORTHINESS

### Data Management

Flip-chart pages were prelabeled with session number and focus, table number, and page number (see Figure 2.4). This system allowed the research team to ensure that data were attributed to the correct session. After each session was complete, flip-chart pages with their sticky note data were removed and taken to a secured room.

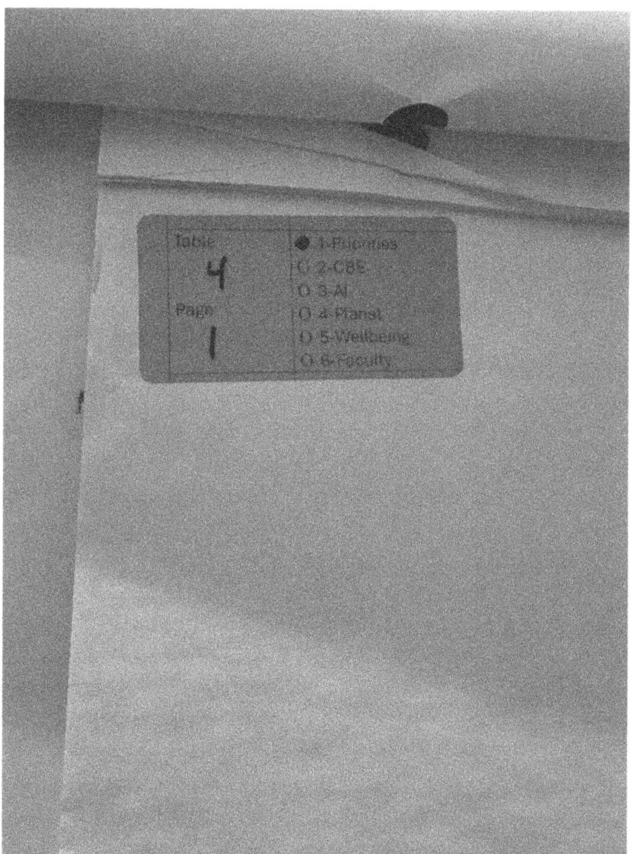


FIGURE 2.4: Prelabeled Flip-Chart Pages

Photographs of each sheet were taken using the Post-it app. Via the Post-it app, the sticky note data were transcribed and exported into an Excel worksheet. The output in the Excel worksheet yielded a copy of each sticky note alongside the transcribed data. Each cell of transcribed data was verified and/or edited for accuracy.

Next, the photographic images of the sticky notes were deleted from the Excel spreadsheet. The Excel spreadsheet then was uploaded to Microsoft Copilot AI. The following prompt was used to export the Excel data into a Word document:

> *Extract the data from the attached Excel spreadsheet and insert into a Word document. Treat the data from each cell as a new paragraph.*

## Data Analysis

Several researchers have deemed AI a legitimate method to conduct qualitative analysis (Hitch, 2024; Maj et al., 2025; Morgan, 2023). For our research, the sticky note data were initially analyzed using NVivo AI and Microsoft Copilot AI to generate themes. The following prompt was used for the session 1 data:

> *Conduct a qualitative analysis on the data from the attached Word document answering the question: What are the educational priorities, strategies, and innovations needed for nursing education and clinical practice by 2030 and beyond?*
>
> *Extract this summary into a Word document.*

The prompt was modified for each subsequent set of data because the table questions changed. The researchers examined the AI-generated themes for face validity.

An Excel spreadsheet was created with data listed in Column A, with each datum on a new row starting on row 2, and themes listed across the subsequent columns for analysis. During Round 1 of data analysis, two researchers (Gillespie, Davis) independently coded each datum against the AI-generated themes. Additional themes were added as needed. Kappa statistics were calculated to identify initial investigator agreement for each datum across each possible theme.

During Round 2 of data analysis, cells without agreement between the two investigators were highlighted. First, Gillespie reviewed the highlighted cells to decide if he would revise his data coding. If he revised the data coding, he edited the cell and removed the highlight. If not, the cell remained highlighted, and he made a notation on the row for his rationale. Davis then reviewed the remaining highlighted cells to decide if she would change her data coding and followed the same process. Kappa statistics were calculated for agreement following Round 2 coding. Finally, during Round 3 of data analysis, the two investigators met to discuss the rationale of their coding and to come to an agreement. A final set of Kappa statistics was calculated. Following Round 3, the Kappa statistics all were 1.000. Table 2.3 lists the Kappa statistics for data from each session.

For activities with voting, frequencies and percentages were calculated based on the number of dots (Gillespie et al., 2025; Mamo et al., 2024). A higher frequency was determined to represent greater importance.

**TABLE 2.3**

**Kappa Statistics for Each Round of Data Analysis**

| Session/Question | Raw Data | Round 1 | | Round 2 | |
|---|---|---|---|---|---|
| | f | f | Kappa | f | Kappa |
| Session 1 | 941 | 883 | 0.918 | 880 | 1.000 |
| Session 2, question 1 | 197 | 197 | 0.890 | 197 | 0.995 |
| Session 2, question 2 | 192 | 189 | 0.861 | 189 | 0.995 |
| Session 2, question 3 | 176 | 165 | 0.937 | 165 | 0.999 |
| Session 3, question 1 | 174 | 170 | 0.906 | 170 | 1.000 |
| Session 3, question 2 | 109 | 106 | 0.875 | 106 | 0.996 |
| Session 3, question 3 | 140 | 140 | 0.819 | 140 | 0.998 |
| Session 4, question 1 | 149 | 147 | 0.930 | 147 | 0.996 |
| Session 4, question 2 | 152 | 146 | 0.903 | 146 | 0.997 |
| Session 4, question 3 | 102 | 98 | 0.871 | 98 | 0.999 |
| Session 5, question 1 | 151 | 143 | 0.846 | 143 | 0.999 |
| Session 5, question 2 | 187 | 182 | 0.881 | 182 | 1.000 |
| Session 5, question 3 | 199 | 193 | 0.879 | 192 | 1.000 |
| Session 6, question 1 | 159 | 148 | 0.926 | 148 | 0.999 |
| Session 6, question 2 | 144 | 137 | 0.907 | 135 | 1.000 |
| Session 6, question 3 | 124 | 119 | 0.903 | 117 | 0.994 |

## Trustworthiness

Trustworthiness of the findings was addressed through credibility, transferability, dependability, and confirmability (Lincoln & Guba, 1985). Credibility was managed through investigator triangulation where the two investigators (Gillespie, Davis) independently analyzed the data and came to an agreement on the findings, as well as peer debriefing with people not included in the project. In addition, member checking of the themes, interpretations, and conclusions was performed with the discussants to address the credibility of the study findings. Transferability was achieved through a thick description of the procedures, context, and description of the discussants (participants). Dependability was addressed by the investigators, creating an audit trail of procedures from generation of the raw data through data synthesis. Confirmability was established by ensuring the findings were grounded in the data. This process can be verified by the generation of Kappa statistics, independent coding (i.e., investigator triangulation), and generation of an audit trail.

## INCORPORATING NLN CORE VALUES

The core values of the NLN are caring, integrity, diversity and inclusion, and excellence. These core values served as guiding principles for the implementation of the Utstein meeting using a World Café method.

### Caring

Although not typically a central tenet of research, caring is a strong core value of the NLN. It was a central tenet in planning the Utstein meeting. Funding was secured to cover expenses (e.g., lodging, coach airfare) for those attendees needing financial support to attend. During the registration process, we asked discussants to note any dietary restrictions or physical/sensory/other accommodations they would need to fully engage in the Utstein meeting. We accommodated all requests. Throughout the meeting, we provided multiple breaks, snacks, and meals. At the end of Day 1, we hosted a reception to allow ample time for discussants and table hosts to network with each other. Following lunch on Day 2, Beverly Malone, president and chief executive officer of the NLN, led a standing ovation in recognition of the catering staff for their welcomeness, food preparation, and outstanding service. We also took time for a group photo to highlight the positive energy being shared during the Utstein meeting (see Figure 2.5).

### Integrity

Integrity, as a hallmark core value of the NLN, as well as research, was ensured through review and approval of the study procedures through formal institutional review board oversight. The World Café procedures adhered to the study protocol. Discussants and table hosts received a letter of information for research prior to the Utstein meeting. The World Café principal investigator (Gillespie) also informed discussants and table hosts about their rights as human subjects prior to the start of the research procedures.

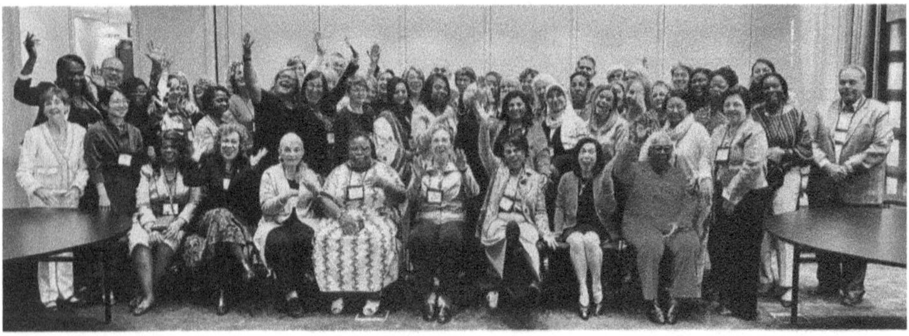

**FIGURE 2.5:** Group Photo of the Utstein Meeting Discussants, Table Hosts, and Support Team

## Diversity and Inclusion

Diversity and inclusion can be actualized in many ways depending on the context. Even though the Utstein meeting was conducted in English, one discussant requested translation services as an accommodation, and these services were provided as requested to ensure the discussant would be included. The discussants represented geographic diversity. The discussants' countries in which they worked spanned 13 countries across all six WHO regions. Their countries varied in income level based on the World Bank categories. Efforts were made to include discussants from low-income countries, unfortunately they were unable to attend due to challenges they experienced with obtaining visas. Finally, table assignments for discussants were randomly preassigned to limit power dynamics that could occur due to ability to speak in English, gender and race dynamics, and communication style. An additional strategy occurred with table hosts managing table dialogues, ensuring each discussant had ample opportunity to communicate their ideas and respond to questions. The member checks that occurred after the Utstein meeting provided another opportunity for people's voices to be heard.

## Excellence

Excellence is the highest level of achievement one should strive for. Our purpose was to strive for excellence with research procedures and with the conduct of the overall meeting. Prior to the Utstein meeting, table hosts were trained in the research procedures and provided written directions. At the start of the Utstein meeting, World Café leaders (Gillespie, Davis) provided refresher training to table hosts and gave them a packet that included the study procedures. Near the end of each round of data collection, table hosts asked discussants to comment on the data that were generated (Azulai et al., 2022). Table hosts then summarized the data to the discussants (Mamo et al., 2024). The meeting and each session started and ended on time. The support team was visible and responsive to individual needs.

## *References*


Albrecht, J., Start, A. L., Dongas, E., Wrona, K. J., & Dockweiler, C. (2022). Hosting an online World Café to develop an understanding of digital health promoting settings from a citizen's perspective—Methodological potentials and challenges. *International Journal of Environmental Research and Public Health*, *19*(9969), 1–19. https://doi.org/10.3390/ijerph19169969

Azulai, A., Tong, H., Quinn, K., & Mykietka, K. (2022). Current and future needs of gerontological social work practice in Alberta: Findings from the World Café at the Gerontological Symposium in Edmonton, Canada. *Journal of Gerontological Social Work*, *65*(8), 832–865. https://doi.org/10.1080/01634372.2022.2047860

Bengtsson, M. (2016). How to plan and perform a qualitative study using content analysis. *NursingPlus Open*, *2*, 8–14. https://doi.org/10.1016/j.npls.2016.01.001

Brown, J., Isaacs, D., & World Café Community. (2005). *The World Café: Shaping our futures through conversations that matter*. Berrett-Koehler Publishers.

Ghafili, A., Azzouzi, W., Hamdoune, M., Gantare, A., Lobet-Maris, C., & Gourdin, M. (2023). Mobilizing the World Café method for adequate development of non-technical skills of midwives in Morocco: A pilot experiment. *Healthcare, 11*(519), 1–10. https://doi.org/10.3390/healthcare11040519

Gillespie, G. L., Meyer, H. A., Bakas, T., & Smith, C. R. (2025). A content analysis defining research-focused faculty success. *Nursing Outlook, 73*(1), 102312. https://doi.org/10.1016/j.outlook.2024.102312

Hitch, D. (2024). Artificial intelligence augmented qualitative analysis: The way of the future? *Qualitative Health Research, 34*(7), 595–606. https://doi.org/10.1177/10497323231217392

Lincoln, Y. S., & Guba, E. G. (1985). *Naturalist inquiry.* SAGE Publications.

Maj, A., Makowska, M., & Sacharczuk, K. (2025). The content analysis used in nursing research and the possibility of including artificial intelligence support: A methodological review. *Applied Nursing Research, 82,* 151919. https://doi.org/10.1016/j.apnr.2025.151919

Maloney, P., & Harper, M. G. (2021). Informing the Nursing Professional Development Scope and Standards: Exploring current and future nursing professional development practice through a World Café methodology. *Journal of Nursing Professional Development, 37*(3), 176–182. https://doi.org/10.1097/NND.0000000000000735

Mamo, N., Tak, L. M., Olde Hartman, T. C., Rosmalen, J. G. M., & Hanssen, D. J. C. (2024). Strategies to improve implementation of collaborative care for functional disorders and persistent somatic symptoms: A qualitative study using a Research World Café design. *Journal of Psychosomatic Research, 181*(111665), 1–8. https://doi.org/10.1016/j.jpsychores.2024.111665

Masse-Grenier, M., Chang, S., Bélanger, A., Stephan, J., Hébert, J., Deschamps, P., Plourde, L., Provost, F., Farzin, H., Fallu, J., Dorval, M., & P3A Research Group. (2024). What do health professional think about implementing psilocybin-assisted therapy in palliative care for existential distress? A World Café qualitative study. *Palliative and Support Care, 22*(5), 1395–1405. https://doi.org/10.1017/S1478951524001494

McConnell, T., Gillespie, K., Potvin, N., Roulston, A., Kirkwood, J., Thomas, D., McCullagh, A., Roche, L., O'Sullivan, M., Binnie, K., Clements-Cortés, A., DiMaio, L., Thompson, Z., Tsiris, G., Radulovic, R., & Graham-Wisener, L. (2024). Developing a best-practice agenda for music therapy research to support informal carers of terminally ill patients pre- and post-death bereavement: A World Café approach. *BMC Palliative Care, 23*(33), 1–15. https://doi.org/10.1186/s12904-024-01369-8

Morgan, D. L. (2023). Exploring the use of artificial intelligence for qualitative data analysis: The case of ChatGPT. *International Journal of Qualitative Methods, 22*, 1–10. https://doi.org/10.1177/16094069231211248

Otto, Q., Nolan, J. P., Chamberlain, D. A., Cummins, R. O., & Soar, J. (2021). Utstein style for emergency care—the first 30 years. *Resuscitation, 163*, 16–25. https://doi.org/10.1016/j.resuscitation.2021.03.022

Rudd, A. D., Bladin, C., Carli, P., De Silva, D. A., Field, T. S., Jauch, E. C., Kudenchuk, P., Kurz, M. W., Laerdal, T., Ong, M. E. H., Panagos, P., Ranta, A., Rutan, C., Sayre, M. R., Schonau, L., Shin, S. D., Waters, D., & Lippert, F. (2020). Utstein recommendation for emergency stroke care. *International Journal of Stroke, 15*(5), 555–564. https://doi.org/10.1177/1747493020915135

Schiele, H., Krummaker, S., Hoffmann, P., & Kowalski, R. (2022). The "research world café" as method of scientific enquiry: Combining rigor with relevance and speed. *Journal of Business Research, 140*, 280–296. https://doi.org/10.1016/j.jbusres.2021.10.075

World Bank Group. (2025). *World Bank country and lending groups*. World Bank Group. https://datahelpdesk.worldbank.org/knowledgebase/articles/906519-world-bank-country-and-lending-groups

Zadvinskis, I. M., Arsenault Knudsen, É. N., Falkenberg Olson, A. C., Eustace, R. W., Albert, N. M., Klein, C. J., Bohr, N. L., Guthrie L. E., & Libster, M. M. (2025). Exploring inclusion by creating inclusion: A World Café among nurse scientists. *Western Journal of Nursing Research, 47*(3), 190–199. https://doi.org/10.1177/01939459241310751

# 3

# Focus Areas for the Future of Nursing Education

**Gordon Lee Gillespie, Sandra Davis, Teresa Shellenbarger, Ilse Wallace, Janice Brewington, Patricia A. Sharpnack, Larry Simmons, Kellie Bryant, Linda Christensen, Yolanda M. VanRiel, and Beverly Malone**

## INTRODUCTION

Nursing is at a pivotal historical point as nursing care delivered in hospital-based settings has begun to decline. In the near future, patients may receive clinical care through alternative care settings, such as telehealth and home hospitals, and by providers such as Amazon Care, Apple, and Google (NCSBN, 2025; Phillips et al., 2025; Weberg, 2021). As health care evolves and incorporates AI, nursing education must radically change, or nursing and nursing education will become irrelevant (NLN AI Strategic Action Group, 2025; Weberg, 2021). To adjust, nursing education must adopt innovations in teaching methods, including simulations, virtual reality (VR), standardized patients, and telehealth (Al Kindi et al., 2025; NCSBN, 2025; Phillips et al., 2025). Recommended curricular innovations include interprofessional education, population-focused care, CBE, informatics, digital technologies, social determinants of health, planetary health, leadership development, and mental health (ICN, 2023; ICN, 2024; NASEM, 2021; NCSBN, 2025; NLN Climate Change and Health Strategic Action Group, 2022; NLN CBE Strategic Action Group, 2023; NLN Social Determinants of Health Strategic Action Group, 2019). In addition, nursing education needs to focus on advanced practice nursing education, faculty shortages, student diversity, and risks of AI in health care (NASEM, 2021; NCSBN, 2025; NLN AI Strategic Action Group, 2025).

## WORLD CAFÉ QUESTIONS

After receiving instructions, Utstein attendees responded to a single question at their respective tables. After predetermined periods of time, they rotated to different tables with new discussants, allowing them to ultimately respond to the same question with different groups. The question was:

- What are the educational priorities, strategies, and innovations needed for nursing education and clinical practice by 2030 and beyond?

This chapter broadly describes the findings based on the discussants' responses to the question about the future of nursing education and highlights the identified educational priorities, recommended implementation strategies, and suggested innovations for the future. Details on the data collection procedures are described in Chapter 2.

# FINDINGS

## Educational Priorities

There are six themes that depict the educational priorities needed for nursing education and clinical practice by 2030 and beyond. The themes are CBE; Digital and Technological Literacy; Inclusion, Equity, and Access; Public and Planetary Health; Nurse and Nursing Faculty Well-Being; and Developing the Faculty Workforce.

### *Competency-Based Education*

Discussants agreed that the future of nursing education should focus on achieving outcomes and building competencies, rather than requiring a minimum number of hours during a clinical rotation. They recommended eliminating time-based measures. Competencies can be developed in collaboration with clinical practice/learning experts and can be individualized with students engaged as partners in their education. Time spent with students can be focused on application, demonstration, and synthesis of competencies. Mastery of skills should be mandatory while still focusing on clinical immersion experiences. Discussants mentioned the terminal outcome associated with CBE; there were multiple recommendations for nursing education to prepare practice-ready nurses for the workforce. However, other discussants suggested that nursing programs must produce nurses who are prepared for clinical practice, not necessarily practice ready, and one discussant requested abolishing practice-ready language altogether. In addition, the discussants mentioned the need for innovative CBE evaluation models. Leaders can standardize metrics to measure nurse quality outcomes and competencies.

### *Digital and Technological Literacy*

The most frequently recommended digital and technological focus for the future of nursing education was AI. Discussants suggested that AI should be integrated into nursing education and that students should be taught about the balance between AI and patient care, AI competency and its risks, and the ethical use of AI. Students should use a critical approach to AI to avoid overreliance and prevent the loss of critical thinking skills. They also recommended that additional new technologies should be incorporated into nursing curricula, such as telehealth, telenursing, nursing informatics, robotics, and machine learning. Electronic health records, technical use of computers, simulation, and augmented reality (AR) are further technologies for curricular inclusion. Technology should be leveraged to ultimately improve patient outcomes. In addition, nurses can serve as developers of digital courses.

### *Inclusion, Equity, and Access*

Discussants indicated that the future of nursing education is one that promotes inclusion, equity, and access for students and faculty coming from diverse backgrounds. Inclusion should focus on diversifying the nursing and faculty workforces, emphasizing cultural diversity, promoting cultural safety, and developing disability-accessible-friendly programs. Discussants also recommended that curricula should be revised to include global competencies on diversity and inclusion and should be multilingual. Finally, nurses should change their narrative and state that all nurses in care roles are important. Equity can focus on eliminating overall bias and bias in assessments. Equity also can be manifested by addressing human rights and ensuring resources for underresourced nursing programs. Access should create pathways for admission, acceleration, and completion of nursing programs. Admission to nursing programs requires eliminating financial barriers for students, which can be addressed by decreasing education costs through technology and government loans for nursing education. In addition, government and philanthropic foundations can invest in nursing education. Access can include the ability of persons in rural and underserved areas to apply to and be admitted into nursing programs. After admission, students need access to tutoring and academic support.

### *Public and Planetary Health*

The discussants suggested that nursing education needs to evolve beyond a focus on acute care nursing in hospital-based settings; it also should include a focus on public and planetary health. They suggested that public health content can focus on primary health care, health and wellness, prevention and public health, pandemics, global health, emergency preparedness, crisis response and recovery, cultural awareness, and public health communication to reduce misinformation. Public health training can occur in virtual home visits, mock disaster drills, and alternative care settings. Public health educational strategies can incorporate recommendations from the European Union's Community Health Strategies and the WHO's Sustainable Development Goals. Planetary health education can include topics such as climate change, global perspectives, reducing medical waste, and how the environment relates to disease.

### *Nurse and Nursing Faculty Well-Being*

Another priority identified for the future of nursing education is the well-being of nurses and nursing faculty. Nurses and nursing faculty need training to promote their personal well-being and to develop self-care skills. Recommendations to accomplish this include education about incivility, implementing student well-being programs, assessing students' mental health, and building resilience. Optimally, interventions will reduce burnout risk; alternatively, nurses and nursing faculty need to learn to work with those experiencing burnout. These interventions are predicated on the ability to create and maintain psychologically safe and healthy work environments.

### *Developing the Faculty Workforce*

A final priority recommended for the future of nursing education is to develop the faculty workforce. Initially, funding is needed for nurse educator programs so that nurses can become faculty and help to address the faculty shortage. The positive aspects of being a nurse educator need to be amplified. To retain faculty, new models of faculty compensation are needed to address the salary gap between nursing faculty and nurses in clinical practice. Discussants suggested that to remain effective faculty need reasonable workloads that include time spent working in clinical practice. Faculty also need continuing education on the use of technology, AI, and interactive and new educational technologies. Funding and resources are needed for self-assessment of faculty competence, faculty and leadership development, and nurse educator certification.

## Strategies for Implementation

There are four themes that depict strategies needed for nursing education and clinical practice by 2030 and beyond. The themes are Interprofessional Education, Collaboration, and Global Impact; Policy and Advocacy Training; Leadership and Career Pathways; and Curriculum Redesign.

### *Interprofessional Education, Collaboration, and Global Impact*

To achieve the future of nursing education, nursing faculty need to work interprofessionally and focus on having a global impact. Health professions education can be incorporated into nursing education to promote interprofessional education. Interprofessional colleagues can support the integration of AI and technology into learning. Interprofessional collaboration can be strengthened through interprofessional research. Nursing programs can collaborate with clinical partners by creating joint appointments. Additional partnerships can be formed beyond the traditional health care systems through private-public and education-regulation partnerships. These partnerships can be leveraged to share technological and other resources. Further, partnerships can be developed with a global mindset. Global partnerships can develop exchange programs between countries to address nurse shortages and address priorities for nurses in partner countries, global health priorities, and advanced practice education. Global partnerships can help to build capacity for all.

### *Policy and Advocacy Training*

Strategies associated with policy and advocacy training emerged. Nursing faculty needs to demonstrate public-policy advocacy and provide advocacy training to nursing students. Faculty demonstrate their policy expertise when they have a presence in the boardroom, strive to remove regulatory barriers to expansion of nursing education, challenge the medical hierarchy, illustrate nursing's autonomy, and practice academic freedom. Public policy and advocacy education for nursing students can include policy and politics, political science, policy development, the art of negotiation, approaches to change, and the importance of involvement in professional associations. In practice, nurses can unionize to have a unified voice as a profession. They need to be represented on national, government, and political decision-making committees. Collective advocacy activities can align policies and regulations in education and clinical practice; eliminate non-evidence-based regulations; recognize nursing as a science, technology, engineering, and mathematics (STEM) discipline; evaluate the impact of policy campaigns on nursing; and remove clinical practice barriers so nurses can practice to the full extent of their education and license. These strategies can compel changes needed for the future and help nurses navigate internal and external political issues and conflicts.

### *Leadership and Career Pathways*

Professional development in leadership and career pathways are needed to advance nursing in the future. Educational content can include systems thinking and complexity, strategic planning and management, leadership skills, political proficiency, generational differences, art of negotiation, finance, and change. Education should be introduced at the entry level to empower nurses to become leaders at the bedside. Career pathways are needed for transitions into nursing, academia, and leadership roles. Early pathway programs can begin by engaging children in nursing school activities to learn about nurses and nursing and then progress to recruiting high school students into health care and nursing careers. Once enrolled in a nursing program, faculty can identify nursing students who show promise in teaching and encourage them to pursue a career as nurse educators. Faculty pipeline development is crucial. Mentorship programs and succession planning are needed for successful faculty development and preparation of diverse academic leaders. Additional strategies recommended by discussants included encouraging lifelong learning, elevating media portrayal and image of nursing careers, and increasing the global brand/image of nursing.

### *Curriculum Redesign*

Another important strategy for the future of nursing education focuses on curriculum redesign. A futuristic curriculum needs to include CBE, nurse entrepreneurship, violence and de-escalation training, conflict resolution, interpersonal and social skills, epidemiology, business and finance, ethics of care, safety and quality, generational conflict, art of negotiation, information overload, social determinants of health and health equity, new technology (e.g., AI), and how to recognize disinformation. Educational strategies to impart this education can include problem-based learning; study-abroad clinical experiences; simulations; teaching using online, hybrid, and blended learning; and educational experiences with underserved populations. Curriculum redesign can be implemented to foster nursing professionals who act with clinical judgment and reasoning and who demonstrate boldness and courage, cultural awareness, humanism, empathy, innovation, and social media competency. In addition, curriculum redesign should include patients and the public and should address environmental issues and pressing public health crises.

## Innovations for the Future

There are five themes that depict the innovations needed for nursing education and clinical practice by 2030 and beyond. The themes are AI-Driven and Personalized Learning, Simulation and Immersive Learning, New Models of Clinical Education, Global Mobility and Standardization, and Advancement of the Science of Nursing and Nursing Education.

### AI-Driven and Personalized Learning

The future of nursing education needs to innovate by incorporating AI and offering personalized learning for students. For education, faculty can leverage AI technology to advance student learning outcomes, clinical competence and judgment, and program efficiency. Faculty can train students on how to integrate AI into clinical practice to reduce errors and advance patient outcomes. Faculty also must train students to use AI ethically while emphasizing humanity and caring. Faculty can use AI to assimilate and synthesize large amounts of student, clinical, and research data. For personalized learning, faculty can incorporate technology into a new CBE-focused curriculum and use data to individualize learning. Technology and AI can optimize AI-driven coaching and self-paced learning, allowing more time for learning in clinical settings. Faculty can further leverage AI for student assessments, development, and remediation to reduce faculty burden.

### Simulation and Immersive Learning

Simulations remain an important innovation for the future of nursing education and clinical practice. Nurse educators in academia and clinical practice can use AI and emerging technologies (e.g., VR, mixed reality, generative AI) to promote immersive learning and augment near-real experiences. Guidelines, clear outcomes, and assessments are needed to help attain simulation goals. Simulations also can be interprofessional and can focus on future error prevention.

### New Models of Clinical Education

Clinical education needs to be revolutionized by incorporating preceptor-based models, developing cost-effective educational models, exploring other pedagogical approaches, changing current assessments, and evolving to keep pace with changes in clinical practice. Students need to graduate ready to practice nursing and spend more time engaged in learning during community rotations. Innovations to accomplish this revolution include incorporating AI, digital skills, and global experiences. Additional clinical education strategies include adopting nursing education models used in other countries, reinventing the clinical nurse specialist role for academic programs, and replacing lectures with strategies such as "TED Talks" so class time can focus on learning activities. In addition, continuing education requirements need to be purposeful and meaningful to advance competencies.

### Global Mobility and Standardization

Nurses and nursing faculty, as global citizens, need the ability to move globally with ethical migration, based on their personal needs, while also addressing nurse and nursing faculty shortages. To be mobile, there needs to be global standards for education and competencies for leadership, defined scope of practice, and clarity of roles. Nurses and nursing faculty need to have a global perspective, be attuned to diversity and inclusion, be aware of global migration, and consider the expansion of the advanced practice role globally. Global mobility can be promoted with degrees that are comparable, portable, and use a common educational language. Nursing education can move toward standardization through accreditation, uniform nurse residency programs, and consistent specialized nursing education programs. In addition, nurse training from high-income countries can be shared with middle- and low-income countries; however, this should be done without excessive influence.

### *Advancement of the Science of Nursing and Nursing Education*

Advancing the science of nursing and nursing education requires innovations in assessment, evidence-based practice, research, training, and entrepreneurship. Components of assessment include improved and diverse evaluation methods, standardization of metrics to measure educational outcomes and nurse competencies, and evaluation of diverse learning modalities (e.g., online, hybrid, simulation). Components of evidence-based practice include monitoring nurse-sensitive outcomes, disseminating best-practice examples, and advancing evidence-based practice grounded in nursing science. Components of research include integrating AI and technology into research; focusing on research priorities from a global perspective; and conducting research on teaching and learning, CBE, evaluation, nursing program effectiveness, and safety and quality. Completing this work requires an investment in educational research. Components of training related to research include teaching students, nurses, and faculty about data generation, processing, and analysis; using evidence to inform education and clinical practice; offering research internships; and preparing nurses to become doctorally prepared nurse scientists who can disseminate research findings on educational best practices and learning behaviors. Components of entrepreneurship include nurses being innovators and visionaries, using technology to invent new technologies, creating new AI and simulations, and recognizing nursing as a STEM discipline. Nursing programs can accelerate entrepreneurship by establishing an innovation center.

## CONCLUSION

Nursing education must evolve to meet the future needs of health care and higher education. Nursing programs need to prioritize education in CBE; digital and technological literacy; inclusion, equity, and access; public and planetary health; nurse and nursing faculty well-being; and the development of the faculty workforce. These priorities require a variety of strategies and innovations such as AI and simulation. To transform nursing education by 2030, nursing faculty and nursing programs will need to examine their curricula through a global and interprofessional lens.

### *References*

Al Kindi, Z., Al Jabri, W., Al Zadjali, M., & Muliira, J. (2025). Utilizing simulation in community health nursing education: A scoping review of current trends and applications. *BMC Nursing, 24,* 1055. https://doi.org/10.1186/s12912-025-03718-1

International Council of Nurses. (2023). *Position statement: Digital health transformation and nursing practice*. International Council of Nurses. https://www.icn.ch/sites/default/files/2023-08/ICN%20Position%20Statement%20Digital%20Health%20FINAL%2030.06_EN.pdf

International Council of Nurses. (2024). *Position statement: Nurses, climate change and health*. International Council of Nurses. https://www.icn.ch/sites/default/files/2024-11/Nurses%20climate%20change%20health%20PS_EN.pdf

National Academies of Sciences, Engineering, and Medicine. (2021). *The future of nursing 2020-2030: Charting a path to achieve health equity*. The National Academies Press. https://doi.org/10.17226/25982

National Council of State Boards of Nursing. (2025). The 2025 NCSBN environmental scan: Going beyond. *Journal of Nursing Regulation*, *15*(4), S1-S48. https://www.journalofnursingregulation.com/article/S2155-8256(25)00038-9/fulltext

National League for Nursing Artificial Intelligence Strategic Action Group. (2025, September). *NLN vision statement: Artificial intelligence (AI) in nursing education*. National League for Nursing. https://www.nln.org/docs/default-source/default-document-library/nln_ai_vision_statement.pdf?sfvrsn=dbb7bef_1

National League for Nursing Climate Change and Health Strategic Action Group. (2022, September). *NLN vision statement: Climate change and health*. National League for Nursing. https://www.nln.org/docs/default-source/default-document-library/vision-series-climate-change-health.pdf?sfvrsn=86ee3340_3

National League for Nursing Competency-Based Education Strategic Action Group. (2023, January). *NLN vision statement: Integrating competency-based education in the nursing curriculum*. National League for Nursing. https://www.nln.org/docs/default-source/default-document-library/vision-series_integrating-competency-based-education-in-the-nursing-curriculum-d6eb0a1e-1f8b-4d60-bc4f-619f5e75b445.pdf?sfvrsn=b37e7538_3

National League for Nursing Social Determinants of Health Strategic Action Group. (2019, April). *NLN vision statement: A vision for integration of the social determinants of health into nursing education curricula*. National League for Nursing. https://www.nln.org/docs/default-source/default-document-library/social-determinants-of-health.pdf?sfvrsn=6078db72_1

Phillips, N., Erickson, J. I., O'Sullivan, H., & Ahmed, S. (2025). The digital future of nursing: Implications for practice. *Nursing Administration Quarterly, 49*(4), 319–325. https://doi.org/10.1097/NAQ.0000000000000694

Weberg, D. (2021, August). *The future of nursing: A paradigm shift moment*. ANA Enterprise. https://www.nursingworld.org/practice-policy/innovation/blog/the-future-of-nursing-a-paradigm-shifting-moment/

PART 2

# Competency-Based Education in Nursing

# 4

# Overview of Competency-Based Education in Nursing

**Jan Jones-Schenk**

CBE is the best solution for nursing education reform to address a challenging history that has included bias and has approached the development of nursing professionals as a game of exclusion rather than inclusion. It is time to put this history and these flawed practices to rest. In the new world of learning, there is opportunity for all and access is not controlled by rigid constraints such as timed pacing. Competency, rather than time, is the appropriate measure for learning.

## THE HISTORY OF TRADITIONAL MEASURES

Credit hours, clinical hours, and grades are long-standing conventions of academic nursing education. The credit hour came from early work to establish a Carnegie unit: a measurable, consistent unit to ensure that educational institutions followed some consistent framework in order to be called a postsecondary university or college (Silva et al., 2015). This unit was defined by time and established in 1906. It was a time in higher education when a type of standard was needed, and time was a thing we knew how to measure. That original metric was defined as the "amount of time a student studies a subject with a teacher." Nothing about learning. Nothing about mastery. In fact, the goal of this original metric was to measure faculty engagement as part of a larger goal to develop a faculty retirement option and sustainable career path. It was also a method for building university budgets. As long ago as the 1960s, this metric was being called into question as a measure of the quality of learning, when it was designed only as a measure of a student's exposure to content. Exposure to content does not ensure or measure learning.

Clinical hours were conceived using the same flawed logic. Hours of time spent being exposed to clinical experiences became a measure for everything from the quality of the nursing program (accreditation) to the requirements for individuals to sit for licensure examination. It is well known there is significant variability in what constitutes a clinical hour and thus its reliability as a measure. Students do not benefit from this definition, which says nothing about learning. In fact, it is the variability in clinical hours that ultimately advanced the adoption of simulation.

Grades, like grade point average (GPA), are false measures that are most often used (and valued) as screens for limiting admission (Jones-Schenk, 2025). For many years, grades have been calculated using a norm-referenced system where the highest "grade" is the one that is the highest in a group of students. Also called "grading on the curve," norm-referenced grading does not measure mastery because the measurement is reflective of what the group "knows" and, in fact, the most knowledgeable person within the group sets the high standard, and a bell curve sets the norm. Grading on a curve means adjusting student scores *after the assessment*. The idea of "the curve" originates with the bell curve. In a typical class, professors can expect a majority of grades to fall near the class average, with a smaller number of A grades and failing grades. Therefore, an A, or 4.0 grade, can mean that the best person in that group knew 70 percent of the material, and the bell curve could easily show a C to mean that 30–40 percent of the material is known by a majority of the students in the norming group. Grades are a statistical distribution of how a group of students perform on a given exam after measurement of the cohort is complete; GPA is an average of those grades. This fuzzy math does not even consider the variability of the quality of the exam and what it purports to measure. Not every exam is well constructed, and many exams have built-in bias and do not actually measure learning. Norm grading is a form of bias. In so many ways our traditional academic metrics are flawed, biased, and do not focus on student outcomes. In higher education, the outcomes of learning should be the most important goal. The ability for students to demonstrate knowledge, skills, and abilities is the most meaningful of outcomes. Grades do not suffice as outcome measures. Even the president of the Carnegie Foundation recognizes the flaws and in 2022 said, "It seems past time to think about how do you build a legitimately outcomes-based system" (Sparks, 2022).

## LEARNING INDIVIDUALIZATION ADVANCES LEARNER ACTIVATION

CBE embraces and addresses the reality that individuals embark on learning and knowing different things at different rates and in very different ways. A second-career nurse with 10 years of experience in accounting may learn at a different pace than a 19-year-old beginning university learner. And even two 19-year-old beginning university learners will likely learn different concepts at different paces based on their prior learning, culture, and personal capacity including socioeconomics and motivations. Starting with the end in mind (competencies) is a different approach than parsing out content a week at a time. It requires a learning environment that is designed to be customized. A key feature of this individualization is that of learner activation. Putting the learner in the driver's seat shifts everything. It also addresses the biases of assumption.

Assumption bias is an unconscious leap to a position or belief based on limited information that may align most closely with what one is used to or comfortable with (Milwee, 2021). In higher education it is systematically imbedded, for example, the assumption that students who perform well on standardized exams are the most capable or those that are more verbal or outgoing in learning settings are more competent or that students who are more "like" faculty or other successful students will be successful. Such biases persist in nursing education and limit the advancement of a nursing workforce that is more reflective of current societal demographics and needs.

Not all confident people are competent, but there is a strong correlation between competence and confidence. Confidence alone is not enough. Kruger and Dunning (1999) identified a phenomenon (the Dunning-Kruger Phenomena) that describes how those who are overconfident in their ability may not actually be the top performers, whereas those who believe they are average, or even slightly below, often demonstrate great skill (Pennycook et al., 2017). This defines something faculty see, and they often praise or value students who are overconfident and project a strong presence or charisma without actual evidence that these students are more competent. Such beliefs are essentially a bias about a student's actual abilities framed by a halo of assumptions (Pennycook et al., 2017). This form of bias can be addressed through CBE and assessment models, thus opening the door for learners who possess capabilities but are limited in their ability to project confidence. The *confidence/competence loop* proposes that if one believes they can do something, they will actually take action to do it, which increases competence and, subsequently, confidence, which spurs the learner to take more action and grow in competence. It supports the idea that all levels of practice are intertwined, so that competence accelerates advancement. It is for this reason that the competence-confidence loop is a critical aspect of learning, particularly in clinical practice.

## THE NATIONAL LEAGUE FOR NURSING CBE DEFINITION

*"CBE holds promise for being able to lift and shift education beyond traditions of credit hours, clinical hours and grades into a new, more fluid future of confident, competent new graduate nurses, at all levels of entry and practice, who will feel prepared and will be prepared to persist in high quality nursing practice across their careers"* (National League for Nursing CBE Strategic Action Group, 2023).

The shift to CBE is a big change that requires commitment, collaboration, coordination, and resources and includes these major elements:

- Students advance upon demonstrated mastery.
- Competencies include explicit, measurable, transferable learning objectives that empower students.
- Assessment is meaningful and a positive learning experience for students.
- Students receive timely, differentiated support based on their individual learning needs.
- Competencies include *application and creation of knowledge*, along with the development of important skills and dispositions.

## THE IMPORTANCE OF ASSESSMENT IN CBE

The most interesting and transformative opportunity to elevate learning in the next century lies in assessments. Learning about the ins and outs of assessments over the past 50 years has revealed many pitfalls and some new opportunities. In recent years, educators may have over-indexed on some aspects of assessment that are not very effective, such as most or all standardized examinations. As educators have developed greater awareness of the pitfalls of bias, limitations, and measurement flaws, it has become clear that assessment requires specific expertise in measurement. Today, simulation is being used for assessment in nursing, something that was frowned on less than a decade ago. What could possibly be more effective in determining the ability of a learner to critically assess and intervene in a clinical scenario than a simulation? There are other improvements to assessment as well. In the United States (U.S.), the licensing examination has been reimagined to focus on the measurement of critical thinking and clinical decision making.

Much has been learned about assessment. Even the mistakes have led to this moment when we can take all that we know, all that we have learned, and apply assessment not as a "one and done" but as a continuous process that engages the learner in self-discovery and self-evaluation. When we "give" grades to students, we foster a passive (and sometimes apathetic) approach to learning. As we begin now to think about measuring competencies through assessment, it becomes apparent that by activating the learner to seek assessment opportunities, the process and ownership of learning is shifted in at least two powerful ways: self-evaluation and reaffirmation of mastery.

1. Two essential underlying professional competencies are self-regulation and accurate self-evaluation. These career-long attributes can be developed as a part of the learning experience. Learners who can become proficient at self-evaluation are lifelong learners and are a huge asset as they advance their competencies across their careers.
2. Creating ways for learners to reaffirm their mastery in multiple ways and multiple times, including on demand, with feedback from multiple evaluators, builds confidence and competence. Both attributes are essential in developing individuals who have career-long commitment and success.

## THE CRITICAL ROLE OF COMPETENCIES IN CBE

In developing competencies for nursing learners, it is useful to consider the full range of complexity that spans the learning process. For example, beginning levels of learning focus more on tasks and content knowledge, but more advanced and higher executive function learning also is built into well-constructed competencies. The CTUS model depicted illustrates the various levels of complexity in defining and assessing competencies: Content Knowledge (C), Task/Skills Knowledge (T), Situated Use of Knowledge (U), and Synthesis and Ethical Comportment of Knowledge (S) (see Figure 4.1). As learners progress in their knowledge, the ways in which that knowledge can and should be used to understand how to best care for patients also advance and change. Knowing how to perform an assessment is one stage of learning, knowing how to probe beyond the obvious or standard of an assessment is a more complex and situated use of knowledge. Knowing how to personalize and apply knowledge to a specific person or the circumstances of that person shows synthesis and ethical comportment of knowledge, its highest and best use.

Critics of CBE have pushed against the model, saying it is only about tasks and is therefore reductionistic. It is only that if we make it that. Competencies that focus on learners' ability to fully assess these key drivers of health and implement strategies to assess and address these drivers of health would make a significant contribution to the

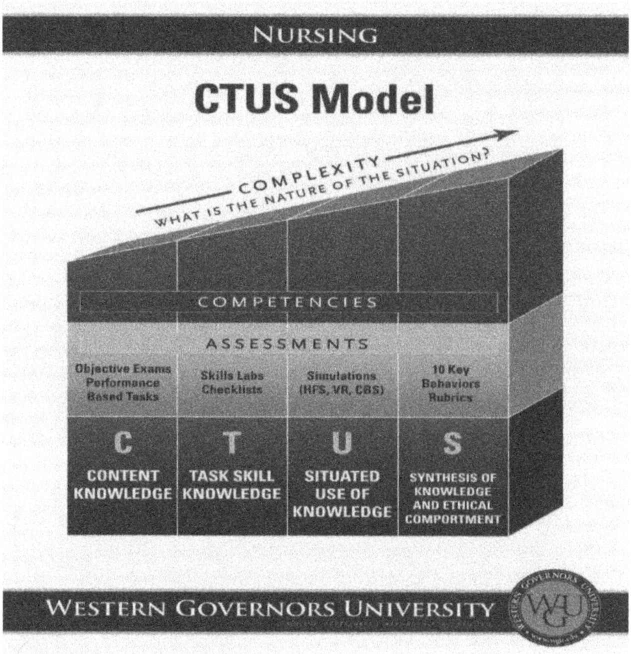


**FIGURE 4.1:** CTUS Model for Competency-Based Nursing Education (Source: Jones-Schenk, 2019)

skills of new nurses and illustrate the higher executive function competencies required for contemporary practice.

Competencies reflect high-level executive functions. The following example reflects how competencies can and should consider complex knowledge, skills, and abilities.

Health and wellness are deeply affected by sleep, nutrition, loneliness, anxiety, and physical inactivity, and these issues are some of the biggest barriers to health that society faces on an individual level. It is well established that sleep is a critical element of health and wellness as well as healing, and while we may teach about sleep, in many cases we have forgotten to emphasize learning how to help people prepare for sleep. However, do we help clients learn how to prepare for sleep in a world of overstimulation that actively works against rest? Do we prioritize rest for our learners, making sure they know that a rested brain and body is more effective and more satisfying?

Loneliness is another particularly intractable health problem. Social isolation is problematic for many groups, including the elderly and underserved populations such as lesbian, gay, bisexual, transgender, and queer (LGBTQ); individuals who are neurodivergent; and any other group that is vulnerable or isolated. Loneliness and social isolation are accompanied by lack of human contact and touch. As nurses, we have long known the power of touch in connection. Touch can be physical or presence. In our driving desire to prepare students with all the content they will ever need to respond to congestive heart failure, diabetes, hypertension, cancer, and a myriad of diseases, do we still teach the importance of connection, trust, and touch? Touch and connection are key to deeply understanding the experiences our clients are having and how they are feeling, reacting, and responding to those experiences, and should be essential competencies for nursing learners. Loneliness and anxiety are strongly linked, often creating a cyclical relationship where one exacerbates the other. Loneliness can lead to increased anxiety, while anxiety can make it harder to form and maintain social connections, leading to feelings of isolation. This connection is bidirectional, meaning that anxiety also can contribute to loneliness. Both problems profoundly affect health, and nursing competencies that address these fundamental human health issues are essential.

Just like this example, if we do not uncover the underlying reasons and values in practice that lie beneath the tasks, we are rightly to blame for a task-oriented approach.

Let us take this example a little further, because it illustrates a potential set of competencies relevant to all populations and nursing care settings. Sleep, rest, connection, and engagement are deep human needs without which there will not be health. That is pretty powerful. An example of a competency that incorporates the knowledge, skills, and abilities necessary to support health behaviors might look something like this:

> *The graduate demonstrates the ability to use a variety of strategies to assess the personal capabilities of the client to implement essential healthy behaviors by assessing knowledge, personal and cultural beliefs, and styles and behaviors to advance client ability to implement new strategies to improve sleep and reduce anxiety for improved health.*

This is a very rough competency statement, which by disclaimer is untested, not peer-reviewed, and not built in collaboration or with assessment preconsideration—all aspects of well-constructed competencies. However, there is still an interesting discussion.

What strategies are needed to assess the personal capabilities of clients? They are far beyond the ability to take a history and physical (H&P). Obtaining an H&P, while an important task, is the most superficial element of client assessment. Although relatively easy to assess, it is incomplete in the case of a competency like this. Knowing how and when to implement touch as a strategy for connecting with a client to elicit trust and deeper communication about issues affecting sleep and anxiety might be one example of a part of this competency, and one that could be assessed through live patient simulation. In fact, simulation is a critical tool for developing and measuring advanced competencies and is the best assessment tool currently available. Computer simulations with unfolding cases can offer excellent opportunities for students to dig deeper and receive feedback on client engagement opportunities that were not fully explored by the learner. Students can try again, with each engagement providing feedback and giving the learner more tools and confidence. In addition, the ability of learners to verbalize the deeper individual challenges a client shares could be assessed through a case study or presentation.

In considering the multilayered aspects of competencies, it is conceivable that this competency, or one like it, might be relevant across multiple courses of study, while the depth of content and assessment differ, becoming more complex as the learner progresses through their program. Competencies like this contain modules of learning that are relevant for all clients, all care settings, and even all caregivers, because learning to manage sleep/rest and anxiety is essential for career-long success as a nurse too!

When my team and I were developing the first competency-based prelicensure BSN nursing program in the United States, we envisioned our graduates as scientists, detectives, and managers of the healing environment. Using this example, the scientists are gaining and expanding knowledge about sleep, anxiety, loneliness, and social isolation, as well as the causes, effects, and potential interventions. The detective is digging under the surface of the H&P and the standard interview to find individualized causation and root cause. The manager of the healing environment is providing feedback, new strategies, and the presence and ability to listen deeply and acutely develop insights required to activate the client to develop new behaviors.

Thinking about assessments across an entire program instead of siloed within a single course is a bit more complex, but also is more effective for the learner and is a best practice in CBE. It also raises the challenging question of how traditional time-bound systems can implement these changes within their systems that have fixed time frames like semesters and fixed requirements like grades. All of this assessment work—the development, alignment, rubrics, grading, and refinement—seems like a lot when we are used to measuring once, when we should be measuring multiple times using multiple methods and multiple people. It clearly requires a shift in how resources are used.

## SPECIALIZATION OF FACULTY ROLES

One aspect that has only begun to receive greater attention in this transition discussion is the evolution of faculty roles to support CBE. Reimagining faculty roles is the best answer to how one might implement CBE within a system still structured around time (Jones-Schenk, 2014). In traditional teaching and learning environments, an individual faculty member does it all. Faculty develop curricula, determine learning objectives and content, deliver content at a paced schedule, create assessments, grade assessments, determine student progression, etc. By unbundling and reconsidering faculty roles, resources can be used differently to better support students and at scale. Faculty also report benefits related to feeling more able to perform in their areas of most competence and in developing new expertise. In a 2021 study of faculty teaching CBE, faculty tended to feel more confident when they could call on their prior experience from teaching in other modalities or from industry. Strong self-efficacy impacts an educator's ability in the learning process (Prokes et al., 2021).

The best competencies are developed in collaboration with clinical practice and learning experts. Developing them is complex because, by definition, they must be relevant and measurable as well as significant enough to support layers of complexity. Like the rough example before, a competency is not a content-linked, time-paced, task-oriented description. Likewise, assessment creation is complex. Learning to develop assessments across a program to measure multiple competencies is a new kind of expertise. It requires collaboration with simulation experts, knowledge of vendor resources and their relevance, and development of new methods to engage learners in self-assessment and peer assessment. This is an expert faculty role that requires focus and relearning. In addition, the assessment expertise must be self-evaluating. It is an important part of this process to make sure that assessments are measuring accurately. Constant evaluation of the effectiveness of assessment tools is essential.

Grading is another area of expertise and is subject to bias, similar to assessment, so the skill set for grading, including the development of rubrics and ongoing monitoring of the efficacy of rubrics for grading, is another area that requires intensive expertise and the attention of faculty experts. Learner individualization and coaching is yet another area of faculty expertise. Using student advancement data, self-evaluation, and advanced coaching skills enables these faculty experts to support individualized learning. Learners then can focus on areas needing development rather than all areas or on areas that the curriculum demands but the learner may not need or may need more of.

While this discussion about evolving faculty roles, including the definition of new areas of faculty expertise, may feel unfamiliar, I point you to the role of simulation educators, which has become such a critical expertise in nursing education. Not every faculty member can be an expert in simulation, so this has evolved to become a specialization. The two areas of assessment and grading expertise will be made even more essential because of the increased use of AI in education. We need these faculty experts to identify the best way to use AI as a tool. In thinking about CBE, simulation, and AI in nursing education, it requires new designs, new skills, new knowledge, and new ways of thinking about teaching and learning.

## THE INTELLECTUAL HUMILITY OF CHANGE

We must collectively embrace our own intellectual humility in order to achieve the dramatic transformation required in learning and teaching. Intellectual humility is the ability to recognize the limitations of one's knowledge and beliefs and to be open to new information and ideas, even if they challenge existing beliefs. In considering the transformation of such an expanse as CBE, it is easy to fall into the trap of simply rearranging or renaming current practices and calling them CBE. Because true CBE challenges so many deeply held beliefs and practices, it may seem so daunting that the easier path, the path of least resistance, is to simply make a few shifts rather than embrace new concepts and recognize one's own limitations of knowledge about an unfamiliar learning model. At this inflection point in learning and in nursing, where the development of the nursing workforce of the future calls us to address the limitations of our current systems, it will be the extent of our intellectual humility and desire to truly reform that will determine whether we advance or stay in our current state. Our belief and confidence in what we know becomes a real barrier to progress and transformation. Our ignorance is invisible to us. Just as it is to our learners. As we seek transformation, we must tune our intellectual humility through curiosity, listening, and gathering new ideas. This is how we will transform nursing education and how we will prepare the nursing workforce of the future to embrace career-long commitment to the profession.

## CONCLUSION

I want to share a passage from an article in *The New Yorker* by D. Graham Burnett, a history teacher at Princeton University, on the topic of AI:

> *"You can no longer make students do the reading or the writing. So, what's left? Only this: give them work they want to do. And help them want to do it. What, again, is education? The non-coercive rearranging of desire"* (Burnett, 2025).

Burnett's comment is equally relevant to the discussion about CBE. In a new world of teaching and learning, the learner is different and will require different things in their learning environment. The desires they bring to the learning environment will demand recognition of their individual needs and abilities, as well as a promise that their learning will be more than a rote, mechanistic, time-bound series of events. CBE focuses on the endpoint. It relies on well-articulated, measurable descriptions of the desired competencies and recognizes that all learners bring unique abilities and learn at their own pace. Unlike the mechanized models of the past, where learning was measured by what could be achieved within a specific time frame, CBE considers that the competency *is* the *standard* and the time it takes is a *learner variable*. That concept reframes how we think about teaching and learning and considers a level of individual support that must be built into systems that may not currently exist. It means that instead of building mounds of curriculum, reading, lectures, and the like, we need to be clear about our competencies and how they will be assessed, so learners will have full transparency and accountability for their outcomes. No more "will this be on the test" moments because what it means to prove competency is transparent and available to all students. Multiple assessments will be needed. The learning is in the process of mastery, NOT mastery itself. Assessments are as critical as competencies, and they must be aligned and developed concurrently. It is truly the growth mindset of learning that has eluded us for so long.

At its highest and best form, CBE places the learner at the center of all decisions. This means that decisions about how learners are treated, tested, communicated with, advanced, evaluated—literally *every* decision related to the learner journey and actual learning—are the first things that are considered (Dana et al., 2021). The structures of the organization must be redesigned with the learner in mind if we are to fully transform higher education to meet the needs of contemporary society.

## References

Burnett, D. G. (2025, April 26). *Will the humanities survive artificial intelligence?* The New Yorker. https://www.newyorker.com/culture/the-weekend-essay/will-the-humanities-survive-artificial-intelligence

Dana, C., Soffe, B., Shipley, J., Licari, F., Larsen, R., Plummer, K., Bybee, S., & Jensen, J. (2021). Why do faculty resist change? *MedEdPublish, 10*, 89. https://doi.org/10.15694/mep.2021.000089.1

Jones-Schenk, J. (2014). Nursing education at Western Governors University: A modern, disruptive approach. *Journal of Professional Nursing, 30*(2), 168–174. https://doi.org/10.1016/j.profnurs.2013.09.005

Jones-Schenk, J. (2019). *Moving toward a competency-based education model [Power Point Slides*]. American Association of Colleges of Nursing. https://www.aacnnursing.org/Portals/0/PDFs/VACN/competency-based-model.pdf

Jones-Schenk, J. (2025). Competency-based education coming to a nursing program near you. *Journal of Continuing Education in Nursing, 56*(1), 8–9. https://doi.org/10.3928/00220124-20241213-03

Kruger, J., & Dunning, D. (1999). Unskilled and unaware of it: How difficulties in recognizing one's own incompetence lead to inflated self-assessments. *Journal of Personality and Social Psychology, 77*(6), 1121-1134. https://doi.org/10.1037/0022-3514.77.6.1121

Milwee, J. (2021). *Unconscious bias: Don't let assumptions influence your decisions*. Women in Localization. https://womeninlocalization.com/unconscious-bias-dont-let-assumptions-influence-your-decisions/

National League for Nursing Competency-Based Education Strategic Action Group. (2023, January). *NLN vision statement: Integrating competency-based education in the nursing curriculum.* National League for Nursing. https://www.nln.org/docs/default-source/default-document-library/vision-series_integrating-competency-based-education-in-the-nursing-curriculum-d6eb0a1e-1f8b-4d60-bc4f-619f5e75b445.pdf?sfvrsn=b37e7538_3

Pennycook, G., Ross, R. M., Koehler, D. J., & Fugelsang, J. A. (2017). Dunning-Kruger effects in reasoning: Theoretical implications of the failure to recognize incompetence. *Psychonomic Bulletin & Review, 24*(6), 1774–1784. https://doi.org/10.3758/s13423-017-1242-7

Prokes, C., Lowenthal, P. R., Snelson, C., & Rice, K. (2021). Faculty views of CBE, self-efficacy, and institutional support: An exploratory study. *The Journal of Competency-Based Education*, *6*, e1263. https://doi.org/10.1002/cbe2.1263

Silva, E., White, T., & Toch, T. (2015). *The Carnegie unit: A century-old standard in a changing education landscape*. Carnegie Foundation. https://www.luminafoundation.org/files/resources/carnegie-unit-report.pdf

Sparks, S. (2022, December 8). *The head of the Carnegie Foundation wants to ditch the Carnegie unit. Here's why*. Education Week. https://www.edweek.org/teaching-learning/the-head-of-the-carnegie-foundation-wants-to-ditch-the-carnegie-unit-heres-why/2022/12

# 5

# Barriers and Strategies for Incorporating Competency-Based Education Into Nursing Education

**Gordon Lee Gillespie and Sandra Davis**

## INTRODUCTION

Competency-based education (CBE) remains an innovative curricular revolution (NLN CBE Strategic Action Group, 2023). It focuses on learners achieving competencies rather than simply passing courses (Atkins et al., 2025; Mani, 2025). Competencies cover a variety of domains including clinical competence, critical thinking, ethics, and interprofessional collaboration (Mani, 2025). Atkins et al. (2025) describe benefits of CBE as academic resources being used more efficiently, students having greater flexibility in the pace of their learning, and students being more prepared to enter clinical practice ready to perform as nurses. They also described that with the efficiencies of CBE, the number of faculty needed could be reduced (Atkins et al., 2025), which, if occurred, would help reduce the burden of the global faculty shortage.

Several challenges impact the ability of faculty to transform nursing curricula. For example, transforming nursing curricula to CBE will require shared terminology (Watson et al., 2026). Any international CBE guideline, including terminology, requires regional adaptations due to varying regulations, ethical frameworks, and culture at the regional to national levels (Watson et al., 2026). Faculty need professional development to lead CBE curricular change, and some faculty may resist this professional development and/or changes to a traditional curriculum (Watson et al., 2026).

## WORLD CAFÉ QUESTIONS

Following a presentation on CBE, Utstein attendees responded to one of three questions at their various tables. After predetermined periods of time, they rotated to different tables, allowing them to ultimately respond to all three questions. The three questions were:

1. What are the barriers and strategies to overcome those barriers to implement CBE globally by 2030?
2. What resources and assessment tools are needed for implementation of CBE?
3. What are the minimum competencies for CBE in nursing?

This chapter describes the findings based on discussants' responses to the three questions on CBE. Details on the data collection procedures are described in Chapter 2.

## FINDINGS

### Barriers to Implementing CBE

There are five themes that depict barriers to implementing CBE globally by 2030. The themes are Faculty-Related Challenges, Structural and Systemic Issues, Resource Constraints, Assessment and Evaluation Gaps, and Globalization and Policy Barriers.

#### *Faculty-Related Challenges*

Faculty-related challenges begin with a lack of awareness at the local, regional, and national levels of what CBE is. Few faculty are formally trained in CBE. Even when awareness is present, there remains a lack of interest, energy, or motivation to transition from the current curriculum to one focused on CBE. On the more extreme side, some faculty are resistant to change. Discussants perceived that these challenges may stem from faculty fears of losing curriculum control, inconsistency over CBE development and implementation, and/or curriculum revision fatigue. Ultimately, global faculty shortage, faculty turnover, and lack of faculty versus student accountability with CBE implementation exacerbate these challenges.

#### *Structural and Systemic Issues*

A key challenge in implementing CBE is the reliance on a medical model within nursing curricula. In addition, various state, provincial, and jurisdictional laws and regulations may influence whether CBE will be permitted as an educational method. Discussants also believed that there is a lack of common definitions for CBE, as well as significant variation with clinical partners, creating further barriers for the implementation of CBE. These issues are confounded by university structures such as a fixed academic calendar, tuition model based on academic credit load, and perceived time needed to revise the curricula and obtain university approval.

### *Resource Constraints*

Financial resources to implement CBE vary by country, which was identified as a common challenge. These financial resources also impact students because the financial aid system is based on academic credit load—students may be unable to secure financial aid to attend nursing school. Further, discussants were concerned about the sustainability of CBE due to evolving health care technologies. Even if these resource constraints were managed, challenges would persist with a lack of funding and time for faculty development on CBE, as well as a lack of CBE experts—albeit discussants only looked inward to their country when stating that experts were not available.

### *Assessment and Evaluation Gaps*

CBE was perceived as too complex to develop competencies and assessments. Even if the tools were available in other countries, assessment tools were not available in most of the discussants' countries. Tools also were not standardized, and there was a perceived lack of research supporting their use. Consistent with previous themes, there were no faculty experts to address CBE competency development, assessment, and evaluation.

### *Globalization and Policy Barriers*

There was a lack of national-level policies addressing CBE in nursing education. Also, there is a perceived resistance to globalizing and implementing CBE. Given the lack of global accreditation standards and lack of CBE community of practice, developing CBE at a global level may not be attainable. There also is the belief that CBE may be too focused on the United States, and other models should be considered.

## Strategies for Implementing CBE

There are five themes that represent strategies to overcome barriers to implementing CBE globally by 2030. The themes are Faculty Development, Policy and Structural Reform, Technology Integration, Engagement of Interested Parties, and Research and Evidence Building.

### *Faculty Development*

Faculty need professional development to become proficient in designing and implementing CBE. This professional development can be standardized and include education on change management. Faculty development can be enhanced by developing a group of CBE leaders/experts who can then provide local training to other faculty members. In addition, the group of CBE leaders/experts can participate in a global faculty exchange program or consortium to diffuse CBE globally. Ultimately, a global certification can be developed and used to identify faculty experts on CBE.

### *Policy and Structural Reform*

First, reform needs to start by exploring clinical and educational models other than the medical model. Second, faculty can adopt a common language for CBE that exists in some countries. Third, local institutional change is needed and can be accomplished by revising faculty assignments, workload, and evaluations; changing clinical placement practices; gaining support from university administrators; incorporating or adapting the traditional academic calendar; and providing incentives to adopt CBE. Finally, faculty can become policy experts and advocate for changes to nursing regulations, state regulations, and accreditation standards, and the adoption of a universal competency framework.

### *Technology Integration*

As technology evolves, faculty can leverage technology, such as simulation, AI, AR, and VR, to implement CBE. Faculty can leverage AI to develop competencies and measurements for CBE. Faculty will need to evaluate emerging technologies in an effort to both implement CBE and to increase the number of students enrolled in nursing programs.

### *Engagement of Interested Parties*

Faculty in nursing programs can partner interprofessionally with other schools and disciplines, such as business, education, and engineering, on technology-based solutions. Sharing resources between schools (within nursing and across disciplines) and clinical practice sites can maximize implementation while potentially reducing costs. Unity is needed across national nursing associations globally to ensure implementation and consistency. In addition, faculty can engage consumers and government entities on the need for and use of CBE in nursing education.

### *Research and Evidence Building*

Scaffolding student assessments across a curriculum is needed and requires the creation of valid and reliable measurements. More outcome measurements need to be relevant to nursing education and based on global competencies, best practices, and standardization of metrics. Research on CBE is needed to determine the scientific basis for these measurements and can be based on a global CBE framework and definitions and student postgraduation outcomes at five years. Establishing a CBE Center of Excellence could promote more evidence-based activities and research on the effectiveness of CBE as a teaching method.

## CBE Resources and Assessment Tools

There are eight themes that describe resources and assessment tools needed for CBE implementation. The themes are Evaluation Methods, Technological Tools, Faculty

Development, Funding, Infrastructure, Policy and Governance, Student Engagement, and Subject Matter Expert/Champion.

### *Evaluation Methods*

Both students and faculty should be evaluated in relation to CBE. Evaluation should be based on a universal definition of CBE and should include portfolios and direct observation of performance. Any rubric, clinical or simulation assessment tool, and checklist-based evaluation should incorporate rubrics and culturally sensitive validated tools that are based on research and established competencies.

### *Technological Tools*

Technological tools for implementing CBE include simulation, AR and VR, computer scenarios, and digital assessment tools. These tools can be leveraged to reduce faculty workload to implement CBE, for example, using AI to aid student assessment. In addition, technology can be used to develop a student dashboard for tracking program and course status.

### *Faculty Development*

Faculty development can take the form of workshops, conferences, webinars, and toolkits. Specific content can include educating faculty on developing computer skills and writing competencies. In addition, faculty can learn how to coach students and teach with interactive methods.

### *Funding*

Funding is crucial for CBE implementation. Financial resources are needed for general CBE resources, purchase of software and AI systems, faculty training and professional development, and research on CBE effectiveness. Because funding is limited, a pragmatic approach should be used for allocation. Key considerations for funding allocation should include hiring more faculty educators, reducing overall faculty workload, and increasing faculty pay.

### *Infrastructure*

Nursing programs' infrastructure needs to be bolstered, which requires an influx of financial resources to develop and support nursing programs as a business. Specific infrastructure components include information technology, CBE platforms, simulation labs, high-fidelity simulators, and student dashboards.

### *Policy and Governance*

Policy and governance occurs at local, regional, and national levels. Locally, nursing programs can increase clinical practice partners' understanding of CBE and offer interprofessional education. Regionally and nationally, faculty can promote regulatory change and review licensure requirements. Globally, faculty can develop faculty exchange programs and global consortiums, competencies, and accreditation standards.

### *Student Engagement*

Students are responsible for their own learning. This responsibility can be strengthened by providing students with individual performance, self-assessment, and peer assessment data. Student learning also should be student-driven and peer-led. To further promote student engagement, faculty can empower students by providing them with tools and resources for learning.

### *Subject Matter Expert/Champion*

A local (school-based) faculty expert is needed to guide CBE implementation. If local experts are not available, schools can tap into the global market for expertise. This need warrants a global expert collaborative to provide CBE consultations and mentoring.

## Minimum Competencies for CBE

There are seven themes that describe minimum competencies for CBE in nursing. The themes are Communication and Interpersonal Skills, Technology and Digital Literacy, Critical Thinking and Decision Making, Clinical and Technical Skills, Ethics and Professionalism, Education and Lifelong Learning, and Leadership and Management.

### *Communication and Interpersonal Skills*

Communication and interpersonal skills are a basic tenet in nursing education for students to learn. Students should be able to demonstrate effective communication and interpersonal skills through therapeutic communication, effective listening, and use of psychosocial skills. Students also should demonstrate empathy, civil discourse, and, when needed, de-escalation. Their ability to communicate with others also can be accomplished with formal presentations.

### *Technology and Digital Literacy*

Technology and digital literacy are routinely needed in nursing practice. Students need to be able to use the technology that delivers health care to advance patient care and outcomes, which may require the integration of AI, as well as how to train AI models. Routinely, students may need to use high-fidelity simulators and student dashboards. Further, students need to demonstrate basic data analytics skills.

### *Critical Thinking and Decision Making*

Students need to be able to use critical thinking to problem-solve and make decisions. They need to be able to use and analyze data to recognize patients in distress and prioritize patient care. Their ability to delegate appropriately and to demonstrate critical thinking and decision making can be validated using CBE.

### *Clinical and Technical Skills*

The clinical and technical skills needed to be demonstrated through CBE include effective technical skills, safety skills, medication administration, and patient education. Students should be able to assess health deficits in patients and identify the need for patient education while addressing science misinformation. They need to be able to provide care while preventing patient and personal injury and reducing risk of illness. They also should be able to promote patient and personal wellness as well as collaborate as part of an interprofessional team.

### *Ethics and Professionalism*

Students should do no harm while practicing ethically and providing person-centered care. They need to model integrity, professional conduct, and the values of a professional nurse. Students need to recognize the difference between ethical and legal aspects of nursing practice. They need to respect their patients' health and human rights. Students need competencies in advocacy, health policy, lobbying, and having a voice in the boardroom. The incorporation of ethics and professionalism can help to form a professional identity and socialization as a nurse.

### *Education and Lifelong Learning*

Students need to have self-insight and reflect on their practice. They need to be committed to lifelong learning and understand how individuals learn. They should base their education on past experiences and seek learning opportunities to apply their future clinical practice.

### *Leadership and Management*

Student competencies in leadership and management can be demonstrated using systems thinking and skills in regulations, logistics and procurement, financial management, strategic planning, organizational leadership, and entrepreneurship. These competencies can help students to further demonstrate the ability to address institutional barriers and enablers, policy, advocacy and systemic changes, and nurse-led solutions.

## CONCLUSION

Similar to the literature, discussants described multiple challenges that can impede the implementation of CBE. These challenges can be overcome through professional development, interprofessional collaboration, and resource allocation. Although discussants recommended globalization of CBE through consortiums and accreditation standards, until some level of agreement can be made on minimum competencies, globalization will be stalled. Further efforts toward globalization will require standardized CBE resources and assessment tools.

## *References*

Atkins, R., Brown, K. M., Mudd, S. S., Ghobadi, K., Baker, D. J., & Szanton, S. (2025). Reimagining nursing education: Leveraging competency-based education, artificial intelligence, and simulation for a diverse and practice-ready workforce. *Nursing Outlook*, *73*, 102582. https://doi.org/10.1016/j.outlook.2025.102582

Mani, Z. A. (2025). Transitioning to competency-based education in nursing: A scoping review of curriculum review and revision strategies. *BMC Nursing*, *24,* 1111. https://doi.org/10.1186/s12912-025-03319-y

National League for Nursing Competency-Based Education Strategic Action Group. (2023, January). *NLN vision statement: Integrating competency-based education in the nursing curriculum.* National League for Nursing. https://www.nln.org/docs/default-source/default-document-library/vision-series_integrating-competency-based-education-in-the-nursing-curriculum-d6eb0a1e-1f8b-4d60-bc4f-619f5e75b445.pdf?sfvrsn=b37e7538_3

Watson, A. L., Bond, C., & Jackson, D. (2026). Competency talk is cheap: Rethinking global standards in nursing education. *Nurse Education Today*, *158,* 106940. https://doi.org/10.1016/j.nedt.2025.106940

PART 3

# Artificial Intelligence

# 6

# Overview of Artificial Intelligence

**Maxim Topaz**

## INTRODUCTION AND BACKGROUND

The integration of AI into health care is rapidly transforming the clinical practice, education, and policy of health care. For nursing education, this shift represents both a critical challenge and an unprecedented opportunity to modernize curricula, prepare future nurse leaders, and ensure inclusive, high-quality care. As the NLN (NLN AI Strategic Action Group, 2025) emphasizes in its 2025 Vision Statement, nursing education must proactively evolve to incorporate foundational knowledge of AI, clinical applications, and ethical considerations—all while addressing challenges in care access and outcomes.

The urgency of this transformation cannot be overstated. AI technologies are already augmenting diagnostic accuracy, patient monitoring, and decision support in clinical settings. The rapid evolution of AI has given rise to groundbreaking tools, including generative language models like ChatGPT, which can generate fluent, coherent text that is nearly indistinguishable from human-produced content (Gosak et al., 2024). As the largest group of health care professionals, nurses are increasingly encountering AI-driven tools in their workflow, which is fundamentally changing their roles and care delivery (Ronquillo et al., 2021). The rise of AI raises ethical and legal considerations, including algorithmic bias and data privacy, as well as the need to ensure that human-centered care is not compromised.

Nurse educators and leaders must proactively prepare the nursing workforce to work effectively and safely with AI. This imperative aligns with the NLN's mission to promote excellence in nursing education, thereby building a strong and diverse nursing workforce that advances the health of our nation and the global community (National League for Nursing, 2025). The NLN implements its mission guided by four dynamic and integrated core values: Caring, Integrity, Diversity and Inclusion, and Excellence. These values must permeate any approach to integrating AI into nursing education, ensuring that technology serves to enhance rather than diminish the humanistic aspects of nursing care.

As health care employers increasingly adopt AI tools, new graduates are expected to work comfortably with these technologies from Day 1. Nursing education leadership recognizes that graduates need to be "AI literate," understanding the capabilities and limits of AI in clinical care. This is fundamentally about patient safety and quality: a nurse who understands how an AI system makes recommendations and its potential pitfalls will be better equipped to use it appropriately, improving patient outcomes.

The success of the nursing process itself is based on the accuracy of nursing diagnoses, which determine nursing interventions and outcomes, and AI can significantly support this documentation process (Gosak et al., 2024).

# THEORETICAL FRAMEWORK: AI LITERACY AND COMPETENCY

## Defining AI Literacy in Nursing

According to Ng et al. (2021), AI literacy involves five key components: knowing, understanding, using, evaluating, and creating with AI. This framework provides a comprehensive approach to developing nursing students' capabilities with AI technologies. Simms (2024) suggests that to successfully incorporate generative AI literacy into nursing curricula, educators should employ a diverse strategy. This involves integrating instruction on AI essentials, covering topics such as machine learning foundations, ethical issues, and real-world health care applications, into current courses like Informatics, Ethics, or Evidence-Based Practice.

The concept of AI literacy extends beyond mere technical knowledge. It encompasses an understanding of how AI systems work, their limitations, and their societal implications. For nursing students, this means developing the ability to critically evaluate AI-generated recommendations, understand the data and algorithms underlying these systems, and recognize potential biases or errors that could impact patient care. As Topaz et al. (2024) note, ChatGPT has the potential to make a significant contribution to the future of nursing education by facilitating learning, promoting improved digital literacy, and fostering critical thinking.

## AI Competency Framework

Chiu et al. (2024) define AI competency as a person's confidence and capability in explaining the workings and societal implications of AI technologies, using them ethically and responsibly, and effectively communicating and collaborating with them in any environment. This definition emphasizes both technical proficiency and ethical awareness, crucial elements for nursing practice.

Russell et al. (2023) identified several essential competencies required for effectively using AI in nursing education and health care. These competencies include:

- Foundational knowledge of AI and its ethical, social, and legal implications
- The ability to evaluate and apply AI tools safely and effectively in clinical practice
- Skills in workflow analysis and practice-based learning
- Capability to engage in the development of AI guidelines and training programs
- Ensuring that AI technologies enhance clinical encounters and contribute to continuous professional development

These competencies aim to promote the safe, ethical, and evidence-based integration of AI in health care. Lattuca et al. (2023) further refined these competencies specifically for nursing education, emphasizing the need for nurses to understand not only how to use AI tools but also how to critically evaluate their outputs and maintain clinical judgment.

### Distinguishing Foundational From Advanced Skills

It is crucial to differentiate between foundational AI knowledge that all nurses need and the more advanced skills required for specialized roles. Foundational knowledge encompasses understanding basic AI concepts, recognizing when AI is utilized in clinical tools, and knowing how to verify AI-generated recommendations. This level of literacy should be universal across all nursing graduates.

Advanced skills, on the other hand, might include the ability to participate in AI system design, conduct algorithmic audits for bias, or lead AI implementation projects. These advanced competencies may be appropriate for graduate-level education or specialized informaticist roles. By establishing this distinction, nursing programs can ensure that all graduates have essential AI literacy while providing pathways for those interested in deeper engagement with these technologies.

## CURRENT STATE OF AI IN NURSING EDUCATION

### Virtual Simulations and Intelligent Tutoring Systems

AI-powered simulation is revolutionizing nursing education by providing more realistic, adaptive learning experiences. As noted by Buchanan et al. (2021), AI-enhanced manikins and virtual avatars can respond to student actions in real time, creating dynamic scenarios that better prepare students for clinical practice. These systems can recognize spoken words, answer questions, and change conditions based on student interventions, making simulations far more interactive than traditional preprogrammed responses.

VR simulations augmented with AI are creating immersive learning environments where students can practice complex clinical scenarios without risk to actual patients. These technologies let nursing students experience rare or high-risk situations that would be difficult to recreate in traditional simulation labs. For instance, AI can dynamically adjust a virtual patient's condition based on the student's assessment and interventions, providing immediate feedback on decision-making skills.

### Adaptive Learning Platforms and ChatGPT Integration

AI-powered interactive learning platforms are revolutionizing the delivery and comprehension of nursing content. These platforms adapt to students' learning pace, preferences, and styles, providing personalized content that enhances engagement and knowledge retention. AlAli et al. (2025) found that these platforms utilize algorithms to analyze student performance data, enabling tailored educational interventions that address individual learning needs and enhance overall competency.

Significantly, generative AI tools such as ChatGPT are now being integrated into nursing education. Gosak et al. (2024) demonstrated that ChatGPT can effectively support the documentation process in nursing education, particularly by helping students identify nursing diagnoses, plan interventions, and specify outcomes according to standardized classifications such as NANDA-I, NOC, and NIC. In the case study, ChatGPT correctly identified content-appropriate diagnoses for a patient scenario, though not all aligned perfectly with NANDA-I classification standards, highlighting both the potential and current limitations of these tools.

## Institutional Case Studies of AI Implementation

Recent case studies from leading nursing schools provide valuable insights into practical AI implementation strategies (Sockolow et al., 2025):

- Drexel University College of Nursing and Health Professions established a 21-member interdisciplinary task force to guide the integration of AI. Their initiatives included developing AI classroom guides with content on literacy, university policies, ethics, and tools for text, image, and video generation. The Education Working Group created faculty resources, including a 10-point checklist for researchers to assess the appropriateness of AI in studies.
- University of Minnesota School of Nursing integrated AI across its curriculum by adding two courses—Database Principles for Healthcare and Data Science for Healthcare—to doctor of nursing practice (DNP) and doctor of philosophy (PhD) programs. These courses teach modern data management and analysis approaches that are conducive to AI use, moving beyond traditional analytical methods, such as Excel, toward approaches more compatible with AI tools.
- The University of Florida College of Nursing established an Office of Artificial Intelligence in 2024 to coordinate strategy, ethics oversight, and technical support. They adopted a tiered integration strategy, aligning with the university's goal of universal AI literacy, and embedded AI content from foundational undergraduate levels to doctoral inquiry.
- Columbia University School of Nursing created streamlined access to clinical data and expertise across campus through their Center for Community-Engaged Health Informatics & Data Science. Their flagship research includes nurse-led early warning systems, home-care decision support, and virtual scribe projects developed in partnership with Columbia's Data Science Institute.

## Assessment and Evaluation Tools

AI is transforming how nursing students are assessed. AI-assisted assessment tools can analyze complex student responses, evaluate clinical reasoning processes, and provide detailed feedback on performance. These tools can identify individual skill gaps and suggest targeted interventions to help students focus on their areas of weakness. By continuously monitoring and assessing student progress, AI helps maintain high educational standards and ensures that graduates are competent and confident in their skills (AlAli et al., 2025).

Natural language processing technologies are being used to evaluate student documentation, ensuring that future nurses develop strong communication skills essential for clinical practice. These systems can analyze nursing notes for completeness, accuracy, and appropriate use of medical terminology, providing immediate feedback that helps students improve their documentation skills.

# CURRICULUM INTEGRATION STRATEGIES

## Didactic Integration Approaches

Integrating AI content into existing nursing curricula requires thoughtful planning and strategic implementation. Many nursing programs are updating their informatics courses to include AI concepts, machine learning basics, and discussions of algorithmic bias. For example, an AI module might be incorporated into a nursing informatics course to introduce types of AI with health care examples and discuss benefits and limitations.

Programs are embedding AI content across multiple courses rather than isolating it in a single class. Evidence-based practice courses now include discussions on how AI can assist in literature searches and synthesis. Ethics courses examine the moral implications of AI-driven decision making in health care. Pharmacology courses might explore how AI systems calculate drug dosing recommendations and the importance of verifying these calculations.

The practical application of generative AI in the curriculum has shown particular promise. Gosak et al. (2024) demonstrated how ChatGPT can be used in nursing education to support documentation of the nursing process. In their approach, students enter patient descriptions into ChatGPT and receive assistance in formulating nursing diagnoses, interventions, and outcomes. Although the tool provided appropriate content-based diagnoses, educators noted the importance of teaching students to verify AI outputs against standardized classifications and maintain critical-thinking skills.

## Simulation and Extended Reality Applications

The integration of AI into simulation education represents one of the most promising areas for innovation. AI-powered simulation platforms can create personalized, adaptive learning experiences based on individual student needs and learning styles. Virtual reality simulations can re-create complex clinical scenarios, enabling students to develop critical-thinking and decision-making skills in a controlled setting.

AR applications are being used to overlay digital information onto physical simulation experiences. For instance, students wearing AR glasses during a physical assessment simulation might see vital sign trends, laboratory values, or AI-generated differential diagnoses displayed in their field of view. This technology enables students to learn how to integrate multiple data sources into their clinical decision making.

Research by Buchanan et al. (2021) suggests that AI-enhanced simulation can significantly enhance learning by tailoring scenarios to learners' needs and enabling simulations of rare or complex situations that are difficult to re-create otherwise. For example, an AI system might generate a patient with a rare genetic disorder, complete with appropriate symptoms, laboratory values, and imaging results, allowing students to practice assessment and management of conditions they might rarely encounter in clinical rotations.

## Generative AI Assignments With Ethical Guidelines

The rise of generative AI tools, such as ChatGPT, presents both opportunities and challenges for nursing education. Rather than prohibiting these tools entirely, progressive nursing programs are developing structured assignments that teach students to use generative AI responsibly. Simms (2024) advocates for a balanced approach that incorporates generative AI literacy into nursing curricula while maintaining academic integrity.

Topaz et al. (2024) suggest that ChatGPT can aid nursing students in writing and structuring assignments by helping them organize thoughts and generate initial ideas. However, they emphasize that clear institutional guidelines and comprehensive education for students on generative AI are essential. For example, students might be assigned to:

- Use ChatGPT to draft a patient education handout, then critically evaluate its accuracy and appropriateness
- Generate nursing care plans with AI assistance, followed by verification against evidence-based sources
- Analyze AI-generated nursing documentation for errors, omissions, or areas of concern

Clear guidelines are crucial for maintaining academic integrity. Syllabi should specify when AI assistance is permitted, require disclosure of AI use, and mandate verification of all AI-generated content against credible sources. Some programs have developed honor codes specific to AI use, requiring students to commit to using these tools ethically and transparently.

## Clinical Education Incorporation

Clinical rotations offer students crucial opportunities to observe and interact with AI systems in real-world health care settings. Faculty can design clinical objectives that specifically address AI competencies, such as observing how nurses utilize clinical decision support systems or analyzing the impact of AI-generated alerts on care decisions.

Students might be assigned to interview practicing nurses about their experiences with AI tools, exploring both benefits and challenges. These conversations can be revisited in postclinical conferences for discussion to help students understand the practical implications of AI in nursing practice. Reflective journals can prompt students to consider questions such as: Did you encounter any computerized prompts or scores this week? How did you and the team respond to them?

Partnerships between academic programs and health care facilities are crucial for exposing students to the latest AI technologies. Clinical sites using AI-powered monitoring systems, predictive analytics platforms, or automated documentation tools can serve as living laboratories where students learn to navigate technology-enhanced practice environments.

## Assessment Strategies

Evaluating student competency with AI necessitates new assessment approaches that surpass traditional testing methods. Rubrics should assess not only knowledge of AI concepts but also students' ability to critically evaluate AI outputs and maintain clinical judgment when using these tools.

Objective structured clinical examinations can be modified to include AI-related scenarios. For instance, a station might present a student with conflicting recommendations between an AI system and clinical guidelines, requiring them to explain their decision-making process and rationale for their chosen action. This type of assessment evaluates both technical knowledge and critical-thinking skills.

Portfolio assessments can document students' growing competency with AI over time. Students may collect examples of assignments where they used AI tools, reflections on clinical experiences with AI systems, and evidence of their ability to critically evaluate AI-generated content. This longitudinal approach provides a more comprehensive view of student development than single-point assessments.

# FACULTY DEVELOPMENT AND INFRASTRUCTURE

## Addressing Faculty Preparation Gaps

One of the primary barriers to effective AI integration in nursing education is inadequate faculty preparation. Many nurse educators lack the technical knowledge, confidence, and experience to effectively incorporate AI tools into their teaching practices. This knowledge gap creates hesitation and resistance to adoption because faculty may feel overwhelmed by rapidly evolving technology.

Case studies from various institutions highlight successful approaches to faculty development (Sockolow et al., 2025). At Drexel University, the task force approach enabled peer dissemination through department and collegewide meetings. The University of Minnesota focused on ensuring faculty were trained or up to date on informatics and AI advances so they could confidently teach students. The University of Florida supported faculty development through collaborations with its Center for Teaching Excellence, including workshops on the use of generative AI in assessment and simulation.

Comprehensive faculty development programs are essential but often lacking. Institutions need to invest in systematic training that addresses both technical skills and pedagogical approaches for teaching with and about AI. This training should be ongoing rather than one time, recognizing that AI technologies and applications continue to evolve rapidly.

## Technical Infrastructure Requirements

Implementing AI technologies in nursing education demands substantial investments in technological infrastructure. This includes not only hardware and software but also robust internet connectivity, cloud computing resources, and technical support staff. Many nursing programs, particularly those in resource-constrained settings, face significant financial limitations that impede their ability to adopt comprehensive AI solutions.

The case studies reveal varied approaches to infrastructure development. The University of Florida's bold AI initiative included an investment exceeding $100 million in AI infrastructure and included the deployment of HiPerGator AI, one of the fastest supercomputers in higher education. In contrast, other institutions, such as Drexel, leveraged existing university resources and volunteer efforts to initiate meaningful AI integration with more limited resources.

Infrastructure requirements extend beyond basic computing resources. Programs need access to AI-enabled learning platforms, simulation software with AI capabilities, and data analytics systems. Licensing costs for these specialized tools can be prohibitive, especially for smaller programs. Additionally, ensuring equitable access for all students, including those who may lack access to personal computers or reliable internet at home, presents ongoing challenges.

## Creating Innovation Ecosystems

To truly embrace AI in nursing education, institutions need to foster a culture of innovation and openness to new technologies. Knighton (2025) suggests that exposure to innovative activities can transform nursing practice and increase the adoption of technological advancements. This requires leadership commitment, resource allocation, and systematic support for experimentation.

Innovation labs or centers can serve as hubs for AI exploration in nursing education. These spaces provide faculty and students with opportunities to experiment with new technologies, develop pilot projects, and share lessons learned. The University of Minnesota's Nursing Knowledge Big Data Science Initiative, now in its 13th year, exemplifies sustained investment in innovation infrastructure.

Interdisciplinary collaboration is particularly valuable. Partnerships between nursing faculty and computer science, data science, and engineering departments can provide nursing faculty with technical expertise, while also giving technology experts insight into health care applications. Columbia University's partnership with its Data Science Institute for developing nurse-led AI projects demonstrates the value of these collaborations.

## Overcoming Resistance to Change

Resistance to AI integration often stems from legitimate concerns about preserving the art and science of nursing. Faculty may worry that increased reliance on technology will diminish the human elements of nursing care or that students will lose critical-thinking skills if they become too dependent on AI tools.

The case studies reveal successful strategies for change management. At Drexel University, involving 21 diverse interested parties in the task force helped build buy-in across the institution. The University of Minnesota's approach of embedding AI concepts into existing courses rather than creating entirely new requirements helped reduce faculty resistance. These examples demonstrate that successful change requires transparent communication about the role of AI as a tool to enhance, rather than replace, human judgment and care.

Professional development also should address the concept of "AI augmentation" rather than replacement. Faculty need to understand that their role remains crucial in developing students' clinical judgment, ethical reasoning, and caring behaviors. Although AI tools can handle routine tasks and provide data analysis, faculty expertise is essential for helping students integrate this information into compassionate, patient-centered care.

# ETHICAL IMPLEMENTATION AND BARRIERS

## Addressing Bias and Misinformation

One of the most pressing ethical challenges in integrating AI into nursing education is addressing inherent biases in AI systems. As Cary et al. (2023) note in their comprehensive review, AI systems can reflect and even amplify biases present in their training data. If an AI risk model was developed primarily on data from one population, it may yield less accurate results for patients of different races, ethnicities, or socioeconomic backgrounds.

This is particularly concerning in nursing education, where fostering culturally competent care is a foundational goal. Students must learn to recognize potential biases in AI outputs and understand how these biases could lead to disparities in care recommendations. For example, an early warning system might miss signs of sepsis in Black patients if the algorithm was trained primarily on data from White patients.

Educators also must address the phenomenon of AI "hallucinations," in which generative AI produces factually incorrect yet convincing content. Gosak et al. (2024) found that while ChatGPT could generate appropriate nursing diagnoses based on patient descriptions, it sometimes produced diagnoses that were not part of the standardized NANDA-I classification, even though it claimed they were. This underscores the critical importance of teaching students to verify AI outputs against reliable, evidence-based sources.

## Academic Integrity Challenges

The availability of generative AI tools raises complex questions about academic integrity in nursing education. Park et al. (2024) highlight concerns about students using AI to complete assignments without developing necessary critical-thinking skills. When learners can effortlessly generate care plans or rationales through AI, they risk bypassing the cognitive processes required for sound clinical judgment and reasoning.

Topaz et al. (2024) note that generative AI can be particularly problematic when students use it to generate text that seems knowledgeable and coherent without truly understanding the content. This could lead to situations where students appear competent in written work but lack the actual understanding necessary for safe clinical practice.

Clear policies are essential for maintaining academic integrity while allowing appropriate use of AI tools. These policies should specify when AI assistance is permitted, require disclosure of AI use, and mandate verification of AI-generated content. Some programs have adopted honor codes specific to AI use, requiring students to commit to using these tools ethically and transparently.

Assessment methods also must evolve to address AI availability. Traditional take-home assignments may need to be redesigned to require demonstration of reasoning processes, not just correct answers. In-class assessments, oral examinations, and practical demonstrations become more important when AI tools can generate written responses. The goal is not to eliminate AI use entirely but to ensure students develop genuine understanding and clinical reasoning skills.

## Resource Constraints and Equity

Implementing AI technologies in nursing education requires significant financial investment, which may exacerbate disparities between well-resourced and underresourced programs. Hostetler et al. (2024) note that infrastructural disparities may limit the effectiveness of AI in underresourced areas, potentially widening educational gaps between institutions with different levels of technological access.

The case studies from Sockolow et al. (2025) illustrate this disparity clearly. While the University of Florida invested over $100 million in AI infrastructure, other institutions, such as Drexel University, relied on volunteer task forces and leveraged existing resources. This variation in resource availability raises ethical concerns about educational equity and whether all nursing graduates are equally prepared for technology-enhanced practice environments.

Solutions require creative approaches to resource sharing and collaboration. Consortia of nursing programs could jointly purchase AI platforms, reducing per-institution costs. Open-source AI tools and educational resources can provide alternatives to expensive commercial products. Government funding and industry partnerships focused on reducing educational disparities can help ensure all nursing students have access to AI education.

## Legal and Accountability Frameworks

The integration of AI in nursing education raises complex legal questions about liability, intellectual property, and data governance. When students use AI tools in their clinical decision making during rotations, questions arise about who is responsible if an AI-generated recommendation leads to an error. Educational institutions must develop clear policies addressing these accountability issues.

Gosak et al. (2024) emphasize that nurses remain licensed professionals and cannot defer responsibility to an algorithm. If AI contributes to a care decision that harms a patient, accountability remains with the health care team. A nurse who administers treatment based on a flawed AI suggestion could still be liable for resulting harm. This underscores the importance of teaching students to treat AI outputs as recommendations, not requirements, and to maintain their independent clinical judgment.

Intellectual property concerns emerge when students use generative AI to complete assignments. Who owns the copyright to AI-assisted work? How should AI contributions be cited? Institutional policies must be aligned with evolving legal frameworks and academic standards.

Data governance becomes critical when AI systems process student information for learning analytics or adaptive education. Institutions must ensure compliance with Family Educational Rights and Privacy Act (FERPA) (when applicable) and other relevant privacy regulations while maintaining systems that are sophisticated enough to provide meaningful educational insights. Transparency about data collection, use, and storage is essential for maintaining student trust.

## Preserving Nursing Values

A fundamental concern in AI integration is ensuring that technology does not compromise the core values of nursing: caring, compassion, and human dignity. The American

Nurses Association (ANA, 2022) emphasizes that appropriate use of AI should support and enhance the core values and ethical obligations of the profession. Any AI implementation that diminishes these values must be avoided.

To preserve these values, careful attention to how AI is presented and integrated into nursing education is required. Technology should be positioned as a tool to augment human caring, not replace it. For example, if AI handles routine documentation tasks, the time saved should be redirected toward patient interaction and therapeutic communication, rather than increasing productivity metrics.

As Topaz et al. (2024) note, the use of generative AI in nursing should not lead to situations where nurses feel less heard or cared for. The technology must align with nursing's ethos of providing compassionate, patient-centered care. Nurse educators must help students understand that although AI can analyze patterns and predict outcomes, it cannot replace human judgment, empathy, or advocacy. These uniquely human qualities remain at the core of nursing practice.

## CALL TO ACTION AND FUTURE DIRECTIONS

The integration of AI into nursing education is not optional; it is imperative. As AI continues to transform health care delivery, nursing education must evolve rapidly to prepare graduates who are not only familiar with AI technologies but also competent in their ethical and effective use. This transformation requires coordinated action from multiple interested parties.

### Recommendations for Nursing Programs

Based on the collective insights from recent research and institutional case studies, nursing program leaders should:

- Establish AI governance committees that include diverse interested parties to guide integration efforts and ensure alignment with educational standards and professional values. The Drexel University model of an interdisciplinary task force provides a successful template.
- Develop comprehensive AI literacy curricula that span from foundational concepts to advanced applications. The University of Minnesota's approach of adding dedicated database and data science courses while embedding AI concepts across existing courses offers a balanced strategy.
- Create clear policies on generative AI use that address academic integrity while promoting innovation. Policies should specify acceptable-use cases, require transparency in the utilization of AI, and establish verification requirements for AI-generated content.
- Invest strategically in infrastructure while exploring innovative solutions to address resource constraints. This includes forming consortia for shared purchasing, leveraging open-source tools, and seeking partnerships with technology companies and other academic departments.
- Prioritize experiential learning with AI tools through simulation, clinical partnerships, and hands-on projects. The University of Florida's tiered integration strategy, spanning from undergraduate to doctoral levels, provides a framework for progressive skill development.

## Faculty Action Items

Faculty must actively engage in professional development to build AI competencies. This includes:

- Participating in training programs, workshops, and collaborative learning communities
- Experimenting with AI tools in their own practice to understand capabilities and limitations
- Modeling responsible AI use and critical evaluation of AI outputs
- Developing new assessment methods that evaluate both AI knowledge and the ability to maintain critical thinking when using these tools
- Contributing to the development of ethical guidelines and best practices for AI in nursing education

## Collaborative Partnerships

Strong partnerships between academic programs and clinical sites are essential for exposing students to real-world AI applications. These partnerships should include:

- Co-creation of learning experiences that incorporate current clinical AI tools
- Shared resources and expertise between academia and practice settings
- Mentorship programs where practicing nurses guide students in appropriate AI use
- Joint research projects that evaluate AI implementation and outcomes

Industry partnerships can provide access to cutting-edge technologies and support for innovation projects. However, these relationships must be carefully managed to ensure educational objectives take precedence over commercial interests.

## Research Priorities

Significant research gaps exist in understanding how to optimally integrate AI into nursing education. Priority areas include:

- Evaluating the effectiveness of different pedagogical approaches for teaching AI concepts
- Assessing the impact of AI education on clinical practice outcomes
- Understanding how AI integration affects the development of clinical judgment and critical-thinking skills
- Investigating strategies to ensure equitable access to AI education across diverse student populations
- Developing validated assessment tools for AI competencies in nursing

## CONCLUSION

The integration of AI into nursing education represents a fundamental shift in how we prepare the next generation of nurses. This transformation extends beyond simply adding new content to curricula—it requires reimagining educational approaches, developing new competencies, and carefully balancing technological advancement with nursing's humanistic values.

The evidence presented in this chapter, drawn from the NLN Vision Statement, institutional case studies, and recent research on generative AI applications, demonstrates that AI has significant potential to enhance nursing education. From personalized learning platforms to AI-supported documentation training, these technologies can improve educational outcomes while preparing students for technology-enhanced clinical environments. However, realizing this potential requires addressing substantial challenges. Faculty preparation gaps must be closed through comprehensive professional development. Infrastructure limitations need creative solutions that ensure equitable access. Ethical concerns about bias, academic integrity, and the preservation of nursing values demand careful attention and clear policies.

The experiences of institutions such as Drexel University, University of Minnesota, University of Florida, and Columbia University show that successful AI integration is achievable through varied approaches adapted to institutional contexts and resources. Whether through volunteer task forces or multimillion-dollar investments, nursing programs can begin meaningful AI integration by starting with clear leadership commitment, interdisciplinary collaboration, and a focus on preserving nursing's core values.

Success in this endeavor demands commitment from all interested parties. Educational institutions must invest resources and create supportive environments for innovation. Faculty must embrace lifelong learning and model critical evaluation of AI tools. Students must develop both technical competencies and the judgment to use AI appropriately. Clinical partners must provide real-world learning opportunities with current technologies.

As we move forward, the nursing profession must maintain its core values while embracing technological innovation. AI should augment human caring, not replace it. Technology should free nurses to spend more time with patients, rather than creating additional administrative burdens. Educational programs that successfully navigate this balance will produce nurses who are both technologically competent and deeply committed to compassionate, patient-centered care.

The future of nursing education lies not in choosing between technology and humanity, but in thoughtfully integrating both to prepare nurses who can leverage AI to improve health outcomes while maintaining the caring relationships that define the nursing profession. Through careful implementation, ongoing evaluation, and unwavering commitment to nursing's values, we can harness AI's potential while preserving what makes nursing unique: the integration of scientific knowledge with human compassion in service to those in need.

### *References*

AlAli, M. F., Qtait, M., Al-Awayssa, R. M., Alquassi, N., & Jaradat, Y. (2025). The impact of artificial intelligence on nursing students: A systematic review. *South Eastern European Journal of Public Health*, *26*(2), 4633. https://doi.org/10.70135/seejph.vi.4633

American Nurses Association. (2022). *The ethical use of artificial intelligence in nursing practice [Position Statement*]. American Nurses Association. https://www.nursingworld.org/globalassets/practiceandpolicy/nursing-excellence/ana-position-statements/the-ethical-use-of-artificial-intelligence-in-nursing-practice_bod-approved-12_20_22.pdf

Buchanan, C., Howitt, M. L., Wilson, R., Booth, R. G., Risling, T., & Bamford, M. (2021). Predicted influences of artificial intelligence on nursing education: Scoping review. *JMIR Nursing*, *4*(1), e23933. https://doi.org/10.2196/23933

Cary, M. P., Zink, A., Wei, S., Olson, A., Yan, M., Senior, R., Bessias, S., Gadhoumi, K., Jean-Pierre, G., Wang, D., Ledbetter, L. S., Economou-Zavlanos, N. J., Obermeyer, Z., & Pencina, M. J. (2023). Mitigating racial and ethnic bias and advancing health equity in clinical algorithms: A scoping review. *Health Affairs*, *42*(10), 1359–1368. https://doi.org/10.1377/hlthaff.2023.00553

Chiu, T. K. F., Ahmad, Z., Ismailov, M., & Sanusi, I. T. (2024). What are artificial intelligence literacy and competency? A comprehensive framework to support them. *Computers and Education Open*, *6*, 100171. https://doi.org/10.1016/j.caeo.2024.100171

Gosak, L., Pruinelli, L., Topaz, M., & Štiglic, G. (2024). The ChatGPT effect and transforming nursing education with generative AI: Discussion paper. *Nurse Education in Practice*, *75*, 103888. https://doi.org/10.1016/j.nepr.2024.103888

Hostetler, T., Owens, J. K., Waldrop, J., Oermann, M. H., & Carter-Templeton, H. (2024). Generative artificial intelligence detectors and accuracy: Implications for nurses. CIN: Computers, Informatics, *Nursing*, *42*(5), 315–319. https://doi.org/10.1097/CIN.0000000000001134

Knighton, S. (2025). Overview and summary: Innovation and design thinking in nursing education and healthcare settings. OJIN: *The Online Journal of Issues in Nursing*, *30*(1), *Overview and Summary*. https://doi.org/10.3912/OJIN.Vol30No01ManOS

Lattuca, M., Maratta, D., Beffert, U., Chevrier, A., & Winer, L. (2023). Healthcare AI: A revised Quebec framework for nursing education. *Quality Advancement in Nursing Education*, *9*(3), Article 2. https://doi.org/10.17483/2368-6669.1408

National League for Nursing. (2025). *Mission and strategic plan*. National League for Nursing. https://www.nln.org/about/about/mission-and-strategic-plan

National League for Nursing Artificial Intelligence Strategic Action Group. (2025). *NLN vision statement: Artificial intelligence (AI) in nursing education*. National League for Nursing. https://www.nln.org/docs/default-source/default-document-library/nln_ai_vision_statement.pdf?sfvrsn=dbb7bef_1

Ng, D. T. K., Leung, J. K. L., Chu, S. K. W., & Qiao, M. S. (2021). Conceptualizing AI literacy: An exploratory review. Computers and Education: *Artificial Intelligence*, *2*, 100041. https://doi.org/10.1016/j.caeai.2021.100041

Park, G. E., Kim, H., & Go, U. R. (2024). Generative artificial intelligence in nursing: A scoping review. *Collegian*, *31*(6), 428–436. https://doi.org/10.1016/j.colegn.2024.10.004

Ronquillo, C. E., Peltonen, L. M., Pruinelli, L., Chu, C. H., Bakken, S., Beduschi, A., Cato, K., Hardiker, N., Junger, A., Michalowski, M., Nyrup, R., Rahimi, S., Reed, D. N., Salakoski, T., Salanterä, S., Walton, N., Weber, P., Wiegand, T., & Topaz, M. (2021). Artificial intelligence in nursing: Priorities and opportunities from an international invitational think-tank of the Nursing and Artificial Intelligence Leadership Collaborative. *Journal of Advanced Nursing*, *77*(9), 3707–3717. https://doi.org/10.1111/jan.14855

Russell, R. G., Lovett Novak, L., Patel, M., Garvey, K. V., Craig, K. J. T., Jackson, G. P., Moore, D., & Miller, B. M. (2023). Competencies for the use of artificial intelligence-based tools by health care professionals. *Academic Medicine*, *98*(3), 348–356. https://doi.org/10.1097/ACM.0000000000004963

Simms, R. C. (2024). Generative artificial intelligence (AI) literacy in nursing education: A crucial call to action. *Nurse Education Today*, *146*, 106544. https://doi.org/10.1016/j.nedt.2024.106544

Sockolow, P., Michalowski, M., Peltonen, L. M., Pruinelli, L., & Topaz, M. (2025). Advancing AI initiatives in nursing academics: Case studies and insights from thought leaders. *Nursing Outlook*, *73*(1), 102527. https://doi.org/10.1016/j.outlook.2025.102527

Topaz, M., Peltonen, L. M., Michalowski, M., Štiglic, G., Ronquillo, C., Pruinelli, L., Song, J., O'Connor, S., Miyagawa, S., & Fukahori, H. (2024). The ChatGPT effect: Nursing education and generative artificial intelligence. *Journal of Nursing Education*, *63*(3), https://doi.org/10.3928/01484834-20240126-01

# 7

# Barriers and Strategies for Incorporating Artificial Intelligence Into Nursing Education

**Gordon Lee Gillespie and Sandra Davis**

## INTRODUCTION

As AI proliferates globally across nursing programs, nursing faculty will find that they need to gauge its utility as a teaching adjunct (NLN AI Strategic Action Group, 2025). The Deakin University School of Nursing and Midwifery in Victoria, Australia, can serve as a model for other nursing programs to develop a curriculum framework for AI literacy (Tomlinson et al., 2026). They embedded and scaffolded AI-focused principles, learning outcomes, and content across their three-year undergraduate program (Tomlinson et al., 2026). Other faculty use generative AI to develop case studies, audiovisual illustrations, quizzes, and guided learning activities (Hamilton et al., 2026). An unclear outcome for AI use is the impact of time needed by faculty. Initially, faculty will need extensive time to learn and train AI systems for incorporation into nursing programs (Hamilton et al., 2026). Notably, the more faculty use AI, the more they become aware of its benefits and risks (Almalki et al., 2025; Saleh et al., 2025).

## WORLD CAFÉ QUESTIONS

Following a presentation on AI, Utstein attendees responded to one of three questions at their various tables. After predetermined periods of time, they rotated to different tables, allowing them to ultimately respond to all three questions. The three questions were:

1. What are the strategies to promote the use of AI in nursing education and clinical practice?
2. What strategies are needed to generate and translate innovative AI teaching and learning practice?
3. What are the challenges and barriers to maintain faculty competence in the rapid evolution of AI?

This chapter describes the findings based on discussants' responses to the three questions on AI. Details on the data collection procedures are described in Chapter 2.

## FINDINGS

### Strategies to Promote AI Use

There are eight themes that depict strategies to promote the use of AI in nursing education and clinical practice. The themes are Faculty Development, Curriculum Integration, Ethics and Guidelines, Interprofessional Collaboration, Technology and Tools, Leadership and Strategy, Equity and Access, and Awareness and Culture.

#### *Faculty Development*

A primary focus incorporating AI into nursing education is faculty development. Initially, an assessment of faculty can occur to identify learning needs as well as dispelling any misconceptions about AI in teaching. This faculty development includes education on how to integrate AI into teaching, training on ethical use, limitations and biases of AI, hands-on learning experiences for faculty, and faculty immersions. Over time, additional training will be needed to refine AI skills and competencies. Additional strategies to promote AI use include developing faculty AI champions and developing an AI microcredential.

#### *Curriculum Integration*

AI needs to be embedded throughout the curriculum so that students develop AI skills. The curriculum needs opportunities for students to have hands-on experiences with AI, such as AI unfolding case studies, simulations, and AI-operated machines. Curricular strands should include learning about AI risks, ethical practices, and creative solutions. To further promote students' ability to develop AI skills, a microcredential can be offered within the curriculum. A benefit of integrating AI into the curriculum is the opportunity for individualized learning pathways; however, discussants identified the risk that students may give up their critical-thinking skills to AI.

### *Ethics and Guidelines*

Clear policies and guidelines need to be developed for AI use, including the parameters for AI use. Key issues include developing data privacy and security guidelines, understanding *who* is missing from AI analyses, and promoting the ethical use of AI. Education on AI ethics needs to be provided to faculty through professional development and through course assignments for students. Policies on academic integrity, privacy, and intellectual property need to be addressed as the use of AI increases. AI ethics discussions, roundtables, and committees can help to create, define, and clarify ethical use of AI. In addition, a legal framework needs to be in place in the event that something goes "bad" with AI use.

### *Interprofessional Collaboration*

Interprofessional collaboration for AI use can begin with academic and clinical practice partnerships. In collaboration with other disciplines, nursing programs can create an AI committee and response team, form an AI legal consultation group, and establish an AI innovation hub. The AI innovation hub could be leveraged to develop new educational strategies with AI experts; host shark tanks with informaticists, engineers, and computer scientists; and develop patient-care robots for home care.

### *Technology and Tools*

AI technology and tools can be leveraged for teaching, informatics, data analysis, patient care plans, electronic health record systems, outcomes assessment (e.g., students, patients), and competency-based learning. To expedite the use of AI, nurses can obtain employment at tech companies and serve on tech company boards. AI is needed to develop patient-care robots, evaluate student assignments, and detect if students used ChatGPT (and other AI platforms) to complete their assignments.

### *Leadership and Strategy*

Nursing program leadership can solicit school, college, and/or university support to allocate funding for AI software and subscriptions, offer incentive grants for AI use, and invest in user-friendly AI systems. Generational differences need to be acknowledged in relation to AI education and adoption. Ultimately, AI use should decrease administrative burden. Higher-level strategies include aligning AI use with accreditation and regulatory bodies, forming national AI nursing commissions, and establishing an AI Center of Excellence program.

### *Equity and Access*

Two major issues with AI use are the high costs that create inequity across nursing programs and the implicit and explicit biases of AI. Although some nursing programs have limited resources to adopt AI technology, the resources could be shared across programs and schools through partnership agreements.

### *Awareness and Culture*

Nursing programs need to consider the value proposition for using AI in nursing education. This value proposition would be enhanced by alleviating fears of AI use, addressing faculty resistance, and identifying AI hallucinations. To promote a culture change, nursing schools or AI experts/champions can showcase examples of early adopter use, promote civil discourse about AI, and explore what role faculty will have in the future.

## Strategies to Generate and Translate AI

There are six themes that describe the strategies needed to generate and translate innovative AI into the practice of teaching and learning. The themes are Faculty Development and Support; Curriculum Integration and Pedagogical Innovation; Ethical, Legal, and Policy Frameworks; Research and Evidence-Based Practice; Technological Infrastructure and Access; and Cultural and Organizational Change.

### *Faculty Development and Support*

Faculty development includes training sessions and sharing successful teaching practices. Training sessions would be enhanced by partnering with clinical practice sites. Additional strategies include peer mentoring, identifying faculty champions, interprofessional collaborations, and AI consortiums.

### *Curriculum Integration and Pedagogical Innovation*

Courses need to be developed or redesigned for curriculum integration based on AI competencies. Content can include education on AI bias and how to query AI to get desired results. AI-generated assignments, rubrics, and assessment tools need to be developed and then evaluated by faculty prior to adoption. Student feedback needs to be incorporated on use and value of assignments generated by AI. Optimally, adaptive learning can be incorporated through AI to provide individualized learning. Diffusion of pedagogical innovations can occur through an AI global learning framework.

### *Ethical, Legal, and Policy Frameworks*

Adoption of AI requires students and faculty to understand the pros and cons of AI use. There needs to be established ethical standards of practice and guidelines for AI use. The use of AI would be further promoted ethically through structures for AI governance, such as accreditation guidelines, regulations, and global standards. Additional considerations for ethical AI use include empowering nursing students to explore AI use and addressing copyright and privacy concerns.

### *Research and Evidence-Based Practice*

The scientific basis for AI use begins with conducting research and encouraging experimentation, which requires research grants and funding. Research studies can test assessment tools and rubrics and new teaching strategies. As data are created, evidence will be generated to establish best practices for teaching and learning.

### *Technological Infrastructure and Access*

Additional faculty are needed to develop and support AI teaching practices. Financial and human resources are needed to overcome barriers to access and use of AI. Specific support includes funding for AI software, validation of AI content, and modernization of nursing labs.

### *Cultural and Organizational Change*

Faculty buy-in is critical to AI adoption in teaching and unifying the language of nursing to support machine learning. Adoption can be enhanced by showcasing early adopters, partnering with clinical practice organizations, creating faculty-learner team competitions, and establishing AI organizational committees. These practices can promote flexibility, change faculty mindsets, and foster a culture of innovation.

## Challenges and Barriers to Maintaining Faculty Competence

There are five themes that describe the challenges and barriers to maintaining faculty competence in the rapid evolution of AI. The themes are Institutional and Structural Barriers, Faculty-Specific Challenges, Pedagogical and Curriculum Concerns, Psychological and Perceptual Barriers, and Strategic and Developmental Needs.

### *Institutional and Structural Barriers*

There is a lack of clear policies at the school and institutional levels, as well as legal and ethical guidelines and frameworks, which inhibit AI faculty competence. In addition, there are concerns about data protection and privacy, intellectual property, rapid change requiring routine updates, access to up-to-date AI, minimal research on AI in nursing education, and institutional commitment. These barriers are further impacted by lack of financial resources, underresourced nursing programs, lack of accreditation standards, and poor internet connection in remote areas where students reside and/or schools are located.

### *Faculty-Specific Challenges*

Faculty do not have adequate peer support, lack access to AI experts, and lack funding for professional development. They have negative beliefs about AI use and posit that the rapid change in AI contributes to information overload, negatively impacting faculty workload. Without clear policies on promotion and tenure, faculty may lack motivation for upskilling. Faculty practice could be further impacted by the risk of losing basic skills after adopting AI use.

### *Pedagogical and Curriculum Concerns*

Incorporating AI into teaching would require changes in the core competencies of teaching, research, and clinical practice. A common framework would need to be developed for a nursing program. Incorporating AI could lead to curriculum overload and a need to manage and control for bias. Without baseline competencies and difference in tools at clinical agencies, the ability to validate competency and understanding would be challenged. In resource-limited environments, nursing programs would have to prioritize which AI tools to adopt. In addition, students may begin to use AI as a "lifeline" for completing assignments.

### *Psychological and Perceptual Barriers*

The use of AI is perceived as "lazy" and increases the risk that students and faculty will lose their basic skills. The inability to manage and control AI bias, lack of consensus on rules and regulations, lack of strategies to address information overload, and proliferation of misinformation and disinformation are significant barriers. Not wanting to say "I don't know" and not knowing who is driving AI developments contribute to faculty fears that they will be replaced by AI.

### *Strategic and Developmental Needs*

Time, resources, and funding are needed to maintain faculty competence with AI. Faculty need to be challenged to become risk-takers and innovators. Setting targets for upskilling and tool learning can help to change the organizational culture. Ineffective change management, lack of infrastructure, and nonsupportive culture contribute to challenges to developing AI for faculty use.

## CONCLUSION

Discussants expressed significant concerns over the adoption of AI in nursing programs as a strategy to enhance teaching and learning. It was believed that adoption would lead to decreased use of critical thinking, loss of skills, and possibly reduced need for faculty to teach students. To continue the proliferation of AI in nursing programs, financial support, organizational commitment, and policies and guidelines on AI use are needed. In addition, ongoing research endeavors are needed to build the science and evidence base for AI use in teaching and clinical practice. Many of the perceived challenges to AI may be overcome by faculty using AI as a resource and experimenting with AI technology and tools.

### *References*

Almalki, M., Sacgaca, L., Pangket, P., Pasay-an, E., Deep, S. H., Maskay, G., Benjamin, L. S., Hashim, S. M. A., Gonzales, A., Rosal, R., Mohsen, M., Mostoles, R., & Lagura, G. A. L. (2025). Integration of artificial intelligence in nursing education: A cross-national exploration. *BMC Nursing, 24*, 1026. https://doi.org/10.1186/s12912-025-03689-3

Hamilton, J., Costello, M., Barr, L., Cooper, S., & Jones, M. (2026). Application of generative artificial intelligence by nurse academics in higher education: A scoping review. *Nurse Education in Practice, 90*, 104669. https://doi.org/10.1016/j.nepr.2025.104669

National League for Nursing Artificial Intelligence Strategic Action Group. (2025,

September). *NLN vision statement: Artificial intelligence (AI) in nursing education*. National League for Nursing. https://www.nln.org/docs/default-source/default-document-library/nln_ai_vision_statement.pdf?sfvrsn=dbb7bef_1

Saleh, Z. T., Rababa, M., Elshatarat, R. A., Alharbi, M., Alhumaidi, B. N., Al-Za'areer, M. S., Jarrad, R. A., Al Niarat, T. F., Almagharbeh, W. T., Al-Sayaghi, K. M., & Fadila, D. E. S. (2025). Exploring faculty perceptions and concerns regarding artificial intelligence Chatbots in nursing education: Potential benefits and limitations. *BMC Nursing, 24*, 440. https://doi.org/10.1186/s12912-025-03082-0

Tomlinson, E., Schoch, M., & McDonall, J. (2026). A curriculum framework for embedding artificial intelligence literacies in pre-registration nursing education. *Nurse Education Today, 158*, 106928. https://doi.org/10.1016/j.nedt.2025.106928

# PART 4

# Planetary Health

# 8

# Overview of Planetary Health

**Teddie Potter**

## INTRODUCTION

Human behaviors are threatening life on this planet. *Homo sapiens*, or modern humans, have walked the earth for nearly 300,000 years (Smithsonian National Museum of Natural History, 2024), and for most of that time our species lived in balance with the rest of nature. However, the recent explosion of the human population, global patterns of increased consumption, and disregard for the well-being of nature have caused massive disruptions to Earth's natural systems (Myers, 2017). These human-caused threats to planetary systems challenge global health and jeopardize the life-support systems necessary for future generations. As the most trusted health professionals, nurses are uniquely positioned to address these challenges. Nursing is grounded in the recognition of interconnection—between individuals, communities, and environments. This chapter contends that planetary health should be a core component of nursing education and clinical practice, reflecting the ethical duty of nurses to safeguard conditions necessary for health and life.

## THE URGENCY OF NOW: MULTI-SYSTEM FAILURE

The health of every individual depends on the effective functioning and interconnection of various systems, such as our cardiovascular, pulmonary, and renal systems. Planet Earth also has interconnected systems or processes that must remain healthy to support life. The Stockholm Resilience Center at the University of Stockholm has determined there are nine planetary processes or boundaries that must not be exceeded if life as we know it is to continue. These boundaries include ocean acidification, biogeochemical flows of phosphorus and nitrogen, freshwater changes, land-use changes, biosphere integrity (loss of biodiversity), climate change, stratospheric ozone depletion, atmospheric aerosol loading (air pollution), and novel entities or synthetic chemicals (Rockström et al., 2009). As of 2023, six of the nine essential boundaries had been exceeded (see Figure 8.1) (Richardson et al., 2023).

The health consequences of climate change are already evident. In the summer of 2022, more than 70,000 people died in Europe due to heat-related causes (Ballester

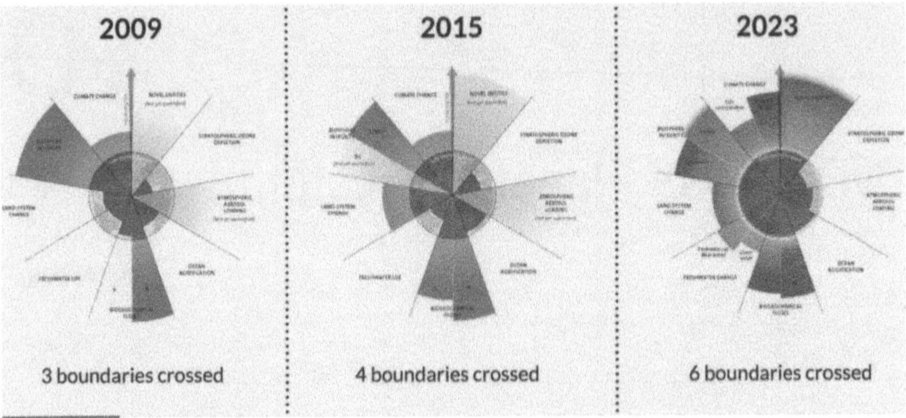


**FIGURE 8.1:** The Evolution of the Planetary Boundaries Framework. (Licensed under CC BY-NC-ND 3.0. Credit: Azote for Stockholm Resilience Centre, Stockholm University. Based on Richardson et al., 2023; Rockström et al., 2009; Steffen et al., 2015)

et al., 2023). Extreme weather events such as the Los Angeles fires in 2025; Hurricane Helene in 2024; and catastrophic flooding in Valencia, Spain, in 2024, and Kerr County, Texas, in 2025 further demonstrate the intensifying threats to human survival. Beyond physical harm, these events compromise mental health and community well-being, increasing rates of anxiety, depression, and trauma (Clayton et al., 2017). Climate change, however, is not the sole ecological challenge; biodiversity loss, pollution, and environmental injustice also threaten health and therefore demand urgent attention from health professionals. How do nurses respond when a patient is in multi-system organ failure? We work with interprofessional teams to restore the physical systems and address the psychosocial and spiritual needs necessary for recovery. The same approach is needed to restore the planet.

## PLANETARY HEALTH: PATHWAY TO A SUSTAINABLE FUTURE

Living sustainably within nature is not new; in fact, most Indigenous cultures have rich values and ethics to help humans live in a right relationship with the land, air, water, and all nonhuman beings. Indigenous values include relationality, reciprocity, and kincentricity, defined as "a view of humans and nature as part of an extended ecological family that shares ancestry and origins" (Martinez et al., 2023, p. 203). Others are beginning to realize that breaking these relationships has serious health consequences. We must learn to challenge harmful narratives and adopt new ways to affirm our interconnection with nature.

In 2015, "Safeguarding human health in the Anthropocene epoch: Report of the Rockefeller Foundation—*Lancet* Commission on planetary health" was published (Whitmee et al., 2015). The report recognizes the interdependence of human health and the health of the planet and that human-caused disruptions to Earth's natural systems are threatening global health. The report is responsible for inspiring the global planetary health movement.

Following the release of the report, the Planetary Health Alliance was launched. The Alliance defines planetary health as "a solutions-oriented, transdisciplinary field and social movement focused on analyzing and addressing the impacts of human disruptions to Earth's natural systems on human health and all life on Earth" (Planetary Health Alliance, n.d.-a). The mission of the Alliance is to:

> Promote, mobilize, and lead an inclusive, transdisciplinary field of Planetary Health and its diverse science, stories, solutions, and communities to achieve the Great Transition, a comprehensive shift in how human beings interact with each other and Nature, in order to secure a livable future for humanity and the rest of life on Earth (Planetary Health Alliance, n.d.-b).

Today, the Alliance represents more than 500 universities and organizations in more than 80 nations (Planetary Health Alliance, n.d.-c), and nurses are active globally.

## PLANETARY HEALTH AS A CORE NURSING RESPONSIBILITY

Nurses are on the frontlines, witnessing the health impacts of environmental degradation. They care for people recovering from disasters and for patients adapting to chronic respiratory and renal diseases related to exposures to wildfire smoke and heat. They listen to patients and communities describe anxiety and despair due to disruptions of livelihoods and housing, as well as threats to the planet and their future.

The ICN (2021) *Code of Ethics* calls nurses to "collaborate and practice to preserve, sustain and protect the natural environment and are aware of the health consequences of environmental degradation, e.g. climate change. They advocate for initiatives that reduce environmentally harmful practices to promote health and wellbeing" (p. 18).

Provision 10.5 of the ANA (2025) *Code of Ethics for Nurses* states:

> Human life and health are profoundly affected by the state of the natural world that surrounds us. Planetary health challenges include environmental degradation, aridification, exploitation of Earth's resources, ecosystem destruction, climate change, waste, microplastics, forever chemicals, and other environmental assaults. These disproportionately affect the health of the poor and ultimately affect the health of all humanity... Nursing brings to the world a uniquely intimate knowledge of the human condition and its interaction with the environment, and is well-positioned to address the social, economic, political, and institutional causes that inhibit health and well-being. (pp. 46-47)

In response to the growing need for nursing involvement, the ICN published *Nursing for Planetary Health and Climate Change,* a topic brief to guide global nursing education and clinical practice (ICN Nursing Student Steering Group & ICN Alliance of Student and Early Career Nurses, 2025). "Nurses should understand how the human caused disruptions to Earth's natural systems (the ecological drivers) impact the health of individuals and communities. Nurses understand the concepts of justice, equity and fairness, and a planetary health lens calls for the extension of these ethical commitments to all species and future generations" (Potter et al., 2025).

In 2025, the ICN Nursing Student Steering Group and ICN Alliance of Student and Early Career Nurses affirmed that planetary health should be embedded in nursing education from the outset, equipping nurses with the knowledge, skills, and confidence to address climate change, ecological disruption, and environmental injustice. Their statement concludes, "Because there is no health without a healthy planet and there is no future of health without the education of nurses who are prepared to protect it. Nurse the planet. Heal the future" (ICN Nursing Student Steering Group & ICN Alliance of Student and Early Career Nurses, 2025). The message is clear—planetary health must become required content in all levels of nursing education.

## WHAT NURSES CAN DO: TEACH, PROTECT, ADVOCATE

Nurses are called to action in three interconnected domains:

1. *Teach the People:* Nurses can educate individuals and communities about environmental exposures, adaptation strategies, and ways to reduce ecological impact.
2. *Protect the People:* Nurses play a vital role in disaster preparedness and response, protecting vulnerable populations during ecological crises. Initiatives such as Community Resilience Hubs demonstrate how nursing leadership can enhance collective capacity for survival and adaptation.
3. *Advocate for the People:* As trusted voices, nurses can influence policy at local, national, and global levels. Advocacy for planetary health aligns with nursing's ethical foundations and extends the profession's commitment to justice. The ICN Nursing Student Steering Group and ICN Alliance of Student and Early Career Nurses (2025) expressed readiness to "learn, lead, and act—grounded in the ethics of our profession and inspired by the vision of a healthy and sustainable world."

## TEACHING PLANETARY HEALTH

To prepare future nurses for these realities, planetary health education must be integrated across curricula. Teaching planetary health is not simply the addition of new content, but rather the creation of a paradigm shift, orienting nursing toward systems thinking, resilience, and ecological responsibility. Teaching planetary health equips nurses not only to recognize environmental determinants of health but also to serve as educators for communities, thereby advancing adaptation strategies and resilience practices.

### Overview

*The Case for Planetary Health* is a short video exploring humanity's impact on the planet and the urgent need for a new path forward (John Hopkins Bloomberg School of Public Health, 2025). The video provides an excellent overview of the planetary health paradigm and why we need to make urgent changes to human behaviors. Following the overview, a deeper dive into the underlying drivers and resulting health impacts is warranted (see Figure 8.2).

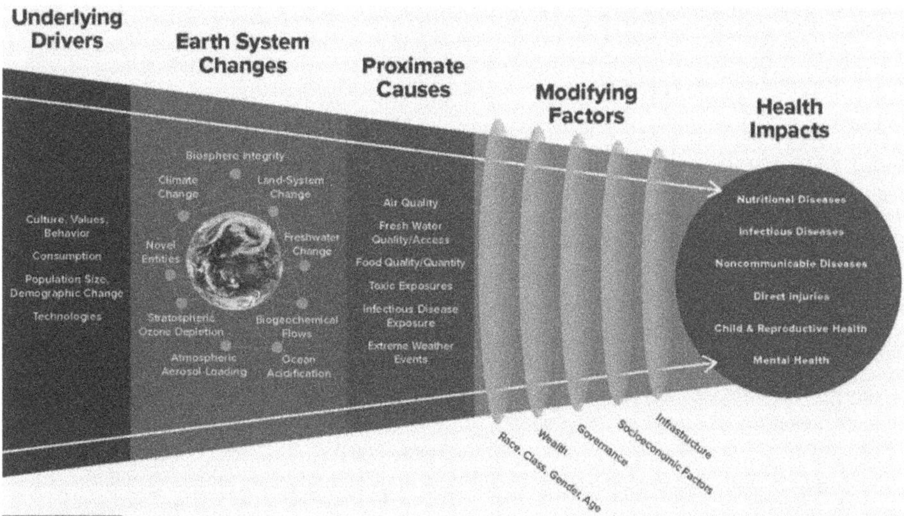


FIGURE 8.2: Planetary Health: Protecting Human Health on a Rapidly Changing Planet. [Graphic modified in 2025 from: Myers, S. S. (2017). Planetary health: Protecting human health on a rapidly changing planet. *The Lancet, 390*(10114), 2860-2868; Duff, H., Faerron Guzmán, C., Almada, A., Golden, C., & Myers, S. (2020). Planetary health case studies: An anthology of solutions. Boston: PHA. https://doi .org/10.5822/phanth9678.]

## Planetary Health Factors

Planetary health curriculum should include a discussion of the cultural values, narratives, and patterns of consumption that drive human behaviors and threaten Earth's natural systems, causing significant changes in Earth systems. These changes lead to proximate disruptions of human health, including poor air quality, the rise of zoonotic diseases, water and food scarcity, and extreme weather events. Eventually, these disruptions result in negative health impacts, including diseases, injuries, and altered reproductive and mental health. It is important to emphasize that social determinants, such as socioeconomic status, race, class, gender, age, education, local policies, and access to care, can disproportionately impact the health of some individuals and communities. Nurse educators need to teach students that nurses can act along the entire continuum; however, addressing the underlying drivers and globally shifting human behavior is the most potent public health action to take.

## Three Essential Planetary Health Resources

Three essential resources to guide planetary health education are *Sao Paulo Declaration on Planetary Health: A Shared Global Vision, Planetary Health Education Framework: A Shared Global Language,* and *Planetary Health Roadmap and Action Plan: A Shared Global Strategy*. Together, they educate students on the principles of planetary health and deliver a vision and strategy for attaining a healthier future.

## Sao Paulo Declaration on Planetary Health: A Shared Global Vision

We are surrounded by evidence that Earth's systems are failing. What is less obvious is that there are reasons for hope. It is therefore essential for students to share a global vision of a possible future in which planetary health is restored. The vision of a future informed by planetary health is found in the *Sao Paulo Declaration on Planetary Health* (Planetary Health Alliance, 2021). The declaration states:

> We need a fundamental shift in how we live on Earth, what we are calling the Great Transition. Achieving the Great Transition will require rapid and deep structural changes across most dimensions of human activity. This includes how we produce and consume food, energy, and manufactured goods; how we construct and live in our cities; and how we consider and measure growth, progress and development, and govern ourselves. It also will require rethinking our values and relationship within Nature and to each other from human exceptionalism, domination, and scarcity to interdependence, equity, and regeneration... We call on governments, the private sector, civil society, and the general public to commit to the Great Transition to safeguard a healthy and equitable future for humanity and protect all life on Earth. (p. 2)

The declaration offers a vision for each sector and a blueprint for transformation. Guidance for health professionals includes:

> Immediately incorporate planetary health concepts and values into the main curricula and professional codes of conduct for all future health practitioners. Educate patients on the concepts of planetary health and utilize health practitioners' trusted voices to raise awareness about the adverse effects of our current dysfunctional relationship with our planet. Draw upon diverse knowledge practices beyond westernized disciplines including those of Indigenous Peoples. Advocate for patient-centered policies that advance planetary health, including public access to health services as a human right, and incorporate solutions and community services beyond the clinic. (p. 6)

The Sao Paulo vision provides nurse educators with a curriculum template to transform global health.

## Planetary Health Education Framework: A Shared Global Language

Although the planetary health field and movements are transdisciplinary, this approach is not customary in academia. Students must be taught to value transdisciplinarity. "Transdisciplinarity complements disciplinary approaches. It occasions the emergence of new data and new interactions from out of the encounter between disciplines. It offers us a new vision of nature and reality" (International Center for Transdisciplinary Research, 1994, Article 3).

To facilitate transdisciplinarity in planetary health, the *Planetary Health Education Framework* (Faerron Guzman & Potter, 2021) was initiated. This framework describes the five core domains necessary to orient higher education students in all disciplines to the planetary health paradigm. These core domains are meant to shape and inform curriculum, and they include:

- Interconnection Within Nature: Humans are inseparable from nature. What we do to nature, we do to ourselves.

- Anthropocene and Health: The planetary health crises are not natural; they are human caused.
- Equity and Social Justice: Solutions must work for all people, not just some.
- Systems Thinking and Complexity: We must address the issues holistically.
- Movement Building and Systems Change: Knowledge is not enough, we must learn to take effective action.

These five core domains act as a shared language that fosters communication and understanding between disciplines. When done well, transdisciplinary engagement fosters new insights and promotes innovative solutions. For example, a nurse, a farmer, and an engineer can work together to design natural and built environments to promote health and sustainability. (See Table 8.1 for a list of planetary health resources.)

## *Planetary Health Roadmap and Action Plan: A Shared Global Strategy*

Strategic planning and highly effective communication will be necessary to collaborate across disciplines to promote the Great Transition to radically shift the upstream drivers of behavior. The *Planetary Health Roadmap and Action Plan* proposes three integrated strategies (Planetary Health Alliance, 2024):

- Reimagine governance institutions fit for the 21st century and beyond,
- Engage the education sector in revolutionizing approaches to education,
- Engage businesses to commit to operating in alignment with planetary health principles (p. 10).

The road map calls educators to embed planetary health content across the curriculum that equips individuals with "up-to-date knowledge, skills, and critical thinking abilities needed to make informed decisions and promote sustainable actions" (p. 13).

| TABLE 8.1 |
|---|
| **Planetary Health Resources** |
| Faerron Guzman, C. A., & Potter, T. (Eds.). (2021). *Planetary health education framework.* Planetary Health Alliance. *https://www.planetaryhealthalliance.org/education-framework* |
| Planetary Health Alliance. (n.d.). *Our health depends on our environment.* Planetary Health Alliance. https://planetaryhealthalliance.org/ |
| Planetary Health Alliance. (2021). *Sao Paulo Declaration on planetary health.* Planetary Health Alliance. https://www.planetaryhealthalliance.org/sao-paulo-declaration |
| Planetary Health Alliance. (2024). *Planetary health roadmap and action plan.* Planetary Health Alliance. *https://planetaryhealthalliance.org/roadmap-action-plan/* |
| United Nations. (2022). *What is the triple planetary crisis?* United Nations. https://unfccc.int/news/what-is-the-triple-planetary-crisis |
| University of Minnesota School of Nursing. (n.d.). *Center for Planetary Health and Environmental Justice overview.* https://nursing.umn.edu/centers/center-planetary-health-and-environmental-justice/center-planetary-health-and-environmental |

## THE PLANETARY LENS IN ALL COURSES AT ALL LEVELS

Promoting a great transition in health might feel daunting, but it really is about inspiring nurses to do what we do best. Based on our holistic understanding of health, human behaviors, and our interconnection with the environment, we think in terms of systems. We also are keenly aware of upstream or underlying drivers. Nurse educators can ensure that environmental determinants of health are considered for every individual patient and every community they serve.

Sustainable practices and decreasing unnecessary waste can be easily threaded into lab courses and clinical practicums, and policies to preserve and restore natural systems can be added to modules on advocacy and leadership. Nurses can be encouraged to work with other health professionals to purchase and use products that have the lowest environmental impacts. For example, the use of single-use products, plastics, and gloves should be evaluated, and decisions made based on science.

Year after year, nursing is consistently recognized as the most ethical profession according to the Gallup Poll (Saad, 2025). Teaching the provisions in our code of ethics is essential for maintaining the public's trust. Addressing threats to planetary health is no longer optional. It is part of nursing's international code and practice. Behaviors required for restoration of planetary health easily align with the core values and ethics of nursing. It is now time for nurses to step forward and lead the efforts toward a sustainable future.

## CALL TO ACTION

The urgency of this moment calls nurses everywhere to embrace planetary health as a professional obligation. Nurses must advance planetary health in health care organizations, communities, and governing bodies, preparing societies to withstand environmental change and fostering hope for future generations. The refrain "Nurse the planet. Heal the future" encapsulates this responsibility and opportunity.

### *References*

American Nurses Association. (2025). *Code of ethics for nurses.* American Nurses Association. https://codeofethics.ana.org/provisions

Ballester, J., Quijal-Zamorano, M., Méndez Turrubiates, R. F., Pegenaute, F., Herrmann, F. R., Robine, J. M., Basagaña, X., Tonne, C., Antó, J. M., & Achebak, H. (2023). Heat-related mortality in Europe during the summer of 2022. *Nature Medicine, 29*(7), 1857–1866. https://doi.org/10.1038/s41591-023-02419-z

Clayton, S., Manning, C., Krygsman, K., & Speiser, M. (2017). *Mental health and our changing climate: Impacts, implications, and guidance.* American Psychological Association and ecoAmerica. https://www.apa.org/news/press/releases/2017/03/mental-health-climate.pdf

Faerron Guzman, C., & Potter, T. (Eds). (2021). *Planetary health education framework.* Planetary Health Alliance. https://planetaryhealthalliance.org/wp-content/uploads/2025/02/The-Planetary-Health-Education-Framework.pdf

International Center for Transdisciplinary Research. (1994). *Charter of transdisciplinarity.* International Center for Transdisciplinary Research. https://ciret-transdisciplinarity.org/chart.php#en

International Council of Nurses. (2021). *The ICN code of ethics for nurses.* International Council of Nurses. https://www.icn.ch/sites/

default/files/2023-06/ICN_Code-of-Ethics _EN_Web.pdf

International Council of Nurses Nursing Student Steering Group & ICN Alliance of Student and Early Career Nurses. (2025). *Planetary health and climate change*. International Council of Nurses. https://www.icn.ch/sites/default/files/2025-05/Planetary%20Health%20SECN%20statement%20-%20EN_0.pdf

John Hopkins Bloomberg School of Public Health. (2025). *The case for planetary health* [Video]. YouTube. https://youtu.be/VUs_2TefNWY?si=I77skMCat6ze_Vv1

Martinez, D. J., Cannon, C., McInturff, A., Alagona, P. S., & Pellow, D. N. (2023). Back to the future: Indigenous relationality, kincentricity and the North American model of wildlife management. *Environmental Science & Policy, 140*, 202–207. https://doi.org/10.1016/j.envsci.2022.12.010

Myers, S. S. (2017). Planetary health: Protecting human health on a rapidly changing planet. *The Lancet, 390*(10114), 2860–2868. https://doi.org/10.1016/S0140-6736(17)32846-5

Planetary Health Alliance. (n.d.-a). *Defining planetary health*. Planetary Health Alliance. https://planetaryhealthalliance.org/what-is-planetary-health/

Planetary Health Alliance. (n.d.-b). *Member organizations across the globe*. Planetary Health Alliance. https://planetaryhealthalliance.org/member-organizations/

Planetary Health Alliance. (n.d.-c). *Our mission*. Planetary Health Alliance. https://planetaryhealthalliance.org/mission-and-values/

Planetary Health Alliance. (2021). *Sao Paulo declaration on planetary health*. Planetary Health Alliance. https://planetaryhealthalliance.org/wp-content/uploads/2025/02/Sao-Paulo-Declaration-on-Planetary-Health-Updated.pdf.

Planetary Health Alliance. (2024). *Planetary health roadmap and action plan*. Planetary Health Alliance. https://planetaryhealthalliance.org/wp-content/uploads/2025/02/Roadmap-to-Planetary-Health-FINAL.pdf

Potter, T., Burton, E., Astle, B., & Honegger Rogers, H. (2025). *Nursing for planetary health and well-being*. International Council of Nurses. https://www.icn.ch/sites/default/files/2025-05/Planetary%20Health%20Topic%20Brief%20-%20EN_0.pdf

Richardson, J., Steffen W., Lucht, W., Bendtsen, J., Cornell, S.E., Donges, J.F., Druke, M., Fetzer, Bala, G., Von Bloh, W., Feuler, G., Fiedler, S., Gerten, G., Gleeson, T., Hofmann, M., Huiskamp, W., Kummu, M., Mohan, C., Nogués-Bravo, D., Petri, S., Porkka, M., Rahmstorf, S., Schaphoff, S., Tobia, A., Virkki, V., Wang-Erlandson, L., Weber, L., & Rockström, J. (2023). Earth beyond six of nine planetary boundaries. *Science Advances, 9*(37), eadh2458. https://doi.org/10.1126/sciadv.adh2458

Rockström, J., Steffen, W., Noone, K., Persson, Å., Chapin, F. S., Lambin, E. F., Lenton, T. M., Scheffer, M., Folke, C., Schellnhuber, H. J., Nykvist, B., De Wit, C. A., Hughes, T., Van der Leeuw, S., Rodhe, H., Sörlin, S., Snyder, P., Costanza, R., Svedin, U., Falkenmark, M., Karlberg, L., Corell, R. W., Fabry, V.J., Hansen, J., Walker, B., Liverman, D., Richardson, K., Crutzen, P., & Foley, J. A. (2009). A safe operating space for humanity. *Nature 461*, 472–475. https://doi.org/10.1038/461472a

Saad, L. (2025). *Americans' ratings of U.S. professions stay historically low*. Gallup News. https://news.gallup.com/poll/655106/americans-ratings-professions-stay-historically-low.aspx

Smithsonian National Museum of Natural History. (2024). *What does it mean to be human?* Smithsonian Institution. https://humanorigins.si.edu/evidence/human-fossils/species/homo-sapiens#:~:text=Species-,Homo%20sapiens,300%2C000%20years%20ago%20to%20present

Steffen, W., Richardson, K., Rockström, J., Cornell, S. E., Fetzer, I., Bennet, E. M., Biggs, R., Carpenter, S. R., de Vries, W., de Wit, C. A., Gerten, D., Heinke, J., Mace, G. M., Persson, L. M., Ramanathan, V., Reyers, B., & Sorlin, S. (2015). Planetary boundaries: Guiding human development on a changing planet. *Science, 347*(6223), 1259855. https://doi.org/10.1126/science.1259855

Whitmee, S., Haines, A., Beyer, C., Boltz, F., Capon, A. G., De Souza Dias, B. F., Ezeh, A., Frumkin, F., Gong, P., Head, P., Horton,

R., Mace, G.M., Marten, R., Myers, S. S., Nishtar, S., Osofsky, S. A., Pattanayak, S. K., Pongsiri, M. J., Romanelli, C., Soucat, A., Vega, J., & Yach, D. (2015). Safeguarding human health in the Anthropocene epoch: Report of the Rockefeller Foundation–Lancet Commission on planetary health. *The Lancet, 386*(10007), 1973–2028. https://doi.org/10.1016/S0140-6736(15)60901-1

# 9

# Barriers and Strategies for Incorporating Planetary Health Constructs Into Nursing Education

**Gordon Lee Gillespie and Sandra Davis**

## INTRODUCTION

Planetary health is evolving as a core construct that nurses need to understand. Nurses in clinical practice are beginning to lead efforts within the health care environment by addressing problems, including sustainable waste management, prescribing practices, and energy-efficient operations (Lokmic-Tomkin et al., 2025). Nursing faculty can impact planetary health by educating students to conduct research and provide advocacy (NLN Climate Change and Health Strategic Action Group, 2022; Vandenberg et al., 2025). However, there is a lack of nursing research on planetary health that can inform education and clinical practice (Vandenberg et al., 2025). Lokmic-Tomkins et al. (2025) explained that integrating planetary health into nursing curricula should be more than adding environmental topics to curricula focused on climate change, which in some countries is a highly politicized topic. Levett-Jones et al. (2025) conducted a Delphi study with 42 international planetary health experts to identify essential knowledge and skills that nurses need. This study resulted in a list of competencies that could be incorporated into nursing curricula. Further, planetary health content can be taught using a variety of teaching methods, including scenario-based learning, simulations, field trips, practice experiences, films, and interprofessional education (Dogan, 2025).

## WORLD CAFÉ QUESTIONS

Following a presentation on planetary health, Utstein attendees responded to one of three questions at their various tables. After predetermined periods of time, they rotated to different tables, allowing them to ultimately respond to all three questions. The three questions were:

1. What are the barriers and proposed solutions for the integration of planetary health into nursing curricula?
2. What strategies can be used by faculty to prepare students to contribute to planetary health research, policy, and advocacy?
3. What is the impact of planetary health on nursing education?

This chapter describes the findings based on discussants' responses to the three questions on planetary health. Details on the data collection procedures are described in Chapter 2.

## FINDINGS

### Barriers to Planetary Health Curriculum Integration

There are five themes that depict the barriers to integrating planetary health into nursing curricula. The themes are Knowledge and Awareness Gaps; Curriculum Constraints; Leadership, Institutional, and Resource Challenges; Political and Systemic Issues; and Cultural and Perceptual Barriers.

#### *Knowledge and Awareness Gaps*

The discussants indicated that, overall, faculty lack understanding and knowledge about planetary health, and there are few faculty experts. In addition, faculty have confusion about what sustainability is. More importantly, faculty do not realize that planetary health is essential to health care and nursing.

#### *Curriculum Constraints*

Undergraduate nursing curricula predominantly focus on acute-care nursing. This one-sided focus was perceived to create inflexible and overloaded curricula. In order to incorporate planetary health content, other courses may need to be eliminated. Current curriculum inadequacies and competing curricular content limit the ability to embed planetary health content.

#### *Leadership, Institutional, and Resource Challenges*

Several challenges were identified. A leadership challenge was the perceived lack of leadership commitment. Institutional challenges were lack of time to revise curricula, faculty reluctance to add the content, and planetary health not being in the school's strategic plan. Resource challenges were lack of funding for faculty development, curricular change, and research.

### *Political and Systemic Issues*

There is a lack of buy-in from students, faculty, nursing programs, and communities for planetary health education. In addition, there are regulatory issues (e.g., minimum clinical hours requirements) and politics of climate issues (e.g., some governments do not support or prohibit planetary health education). Another political issue is that middle- and low-income countries want to industrialize similar to high-income countries.

### *Cultural and Perceptual Barriers*

Faculty lack of buy-in that planetary health is a problem serves as a perceptual barrier. For some faculty, planetary health may be important but just not as important as other topics. Other barriers include planetary health being too upstream for a nursing focus, a perception that nothing can be done, and the perception that planetary health does not affect them. In addition, faculty are unclear about what students would do with planetary health content. Culturally, a focus on planetary health (e.g., recycling) was believed to not happen in rural communities and therefore not be relevant for nursing programs.

## Proposed Solutions for Planetary Health Curriculum Integration

There are six themes that depict the proposed solutions for integrating planetary health into nursing curricula. The themes are Faculty Development and Training, Curriculum Integration, Policy and Accreditation, Student Engagement, Interprofessional and Community Approaches, and Strategic Communication and Framing.

### *Faculty Development and Training*

Faculty need professional development and training on planetary health. This content can be delivered via workshops, conferences, and microcourses. Funding is needed for this professional development. Additional strategies include appointing a faculty champion or change agent and asking faculty to examine their own behaviors regarding planetary health.

### *Curriculum Integration*

Rather than offering planetary health as a stand-alone course, discussants recommend that content be integrated throughout the curriculum. The content could become a program requirement embedded within a policy, community, or public health course and/or a compulsory module in another course. In order to accommodate planetary health into the curriculum, faculty could review the curriculum and eliminate some courses, include planetary health within a community health certification, and increase non-hospital clinicals to 80 percent of clinical practice hours. The school, college, and/or university also could offer faculty incentive grants to incorporate planetary health into courses.

### *Policy and Accreditation*

The diffusion of planetary health content can be enhanced through policy regulation, accreditation criteria, and nursing dean commitment. Additional strategies to support curricular efforts include nursing licensure examinations, including planetary health-related questions, government commitment to planetary health, national nursing associations prioritizing planetary health, world vision on planetary health, and promoting the NLN Center of Excellence for Creating Learning Environments that Impact Climate Change and Planetary Health.

### *Student Engagement*

Students can engage in planetary health by first examining their own behaviors. Next, students can join student-focused interest groups and perform public-policy advocacy for planetary health. Later, students can conduct undergraduate projects, clinical doctorate (i.e., doctor of nursing practice) scholarly projects, and research doctorate (i.e., doctor of philosophy) dissertations focused on planetary health. Finally, students can advocate for curricular change.

### *Interprofessional and Community Approaches*

Nursing is a trusted resource to communities, which can be leveraged to partner with community leaders and Indigenous peoples to address planetary health at the community level. Faculty can collaborate with other disciplines for disaster preparedness and planetary health research. Nurses and nursing faculty also can volunteer at disaster sites and join planetary health-focused professional associations.

### *Strategic Communication and Framing*

A unifying narrative is needed to create the imperative for planetary health education. This narrative needs to be aware of politics and consider that some words are politically charged. In addition, faculty need to create space for uncomfortable conversations and highlight the link between planetary health and social justice and equity. These efforts can emphasize nursing ethics and values. Faculty also can share examples of solutions that nurses have implemented and create case examples about impact. Importantly, faculty need to role model what they teach about planetary health.

## Strategies to Prepare Students to Make a Contribution

There are seven themes that convey strategies that faculty can use to prepare students to contribute to planetary health research, policy, and advocacy. The themes are Curriculum Integration and Development, Faculty Preparation and Leadership, Student Engagement and Empowerment, Research and Scholarly Activity, Policy and Advocacy Training, Interprofessional and Community Collaboration, and Innovation and Resource Mobilization.

### Curriculum Integration and Development

As the curriculum is revised to incorporate planetary health, it can use a planet to society to community to family to individual framework. It also should be taught across the curriculum to achieve a variety of planetary health competencies. For example, content can be embedded within simulations; patient, family, and neighborhood assessments; and internship experiences. Specific recommendations for content include social determinants of health, biomedical hazards, supplies used for patient care and medical waste, disaster management, and ethical issues and values. Planetary health education can prepare students for public health advocacy and to obtain community and public health careers. Importantly, faculty need to serve as role models.

### Faculty Preparation and Leadership

To serve as role models, faculty must start with professional development on planetary health. As their expertise increases, they can become faculty champions. This need for faculty development, role modeling, and appointing faculty champions was mentioned multiple times by the discussants.

### Student Engagement and Empowerment

For students to become better engaged in planetary health, they can start by becoming more aware of their personal activities and reducing waste. They also can join student clubs and groups and participate in regular activities and planetary health forums. Students also can participate in student exchange programs with countries more greatly impacted by planetary health and can complete coursework that prepares them for advocacy.

### Research and Scholarly Activity

Locally, students can lead projects focused on planetary health from the undergraduate level to doctoral levels (i.e., doctor of nursing practice scholarly projects, doctor of philosophy dissertations). Students can complete their projects individually or in groups. Nationally, research funding should be made available through national agencies (e.g., U.S. National Institute for Nursing Research, U.S. National Institute of Environmental Health Sciences). To support research and scholarly activities, faculty can serve as advisers and dissertation chairs, incorporate community projects in the courses they teach, conduct research relevant to disasters, and monitor and evaluate integration.

### Policy and Advocacy Training

Students can participate in policy and advocacy training by taking coursework focused on public-policy advocacy, using environmentally focused bills for health policy assignments, and attending city/local council meetings. Faculty can incorporate environmental health policy into their courses and mentor students to conduct public-policy advocacy. Nursing programs can adopt a policy that shows its commitment to planetary health. Nationally, accrediting bodies can incorporate planetary health into their accreditation criteria. At all levels, nurses and nursing faculty can strive to depoliticize the topic of planetary health, link students and nurses to local government resources, and elect nurses to the legislature.

### *Interprofessional and Community Collaboration*

Students and faculty need to collaborate with other disciplines for coursework and community activities. Faculty also can partner with the local community, nursing schools in other countries, and professional associations. Students can join their national student nurses' association and steer the association to be active in planetary health. Faculty can join associations focused on planetary health.

### *Innovation and Resource Mobilization*

Mobilization of resources can occur through campaigns to engage health care organizations in planetary health. Financial resources are needed to support students and faculty in conducting planetary health projects. Social media can be leveraged to raise awareness and celebrate Earth Day (April 22nd each year) and similar days.

## Impact of Planetary Health on Nursing Education

There are five themes that depict the impact of planetary health on nursing education. The themes are Environmental and Health Awareness, Curriculum Integration, Faculty Development, Innovation and Change, and Challenges and Barriers.

### *Environmental and Health Awareness*

The impact of planetary health necessitates that students not only have a strong understanding of it but also be able to apply systems thinking, think globally versus locally, be sensitive to resource use, and embrace planetary health as a value. Nursing education needs to provide opportunities for faculty and students to collaborate with other agencies, promote prevention strategies, and address disaster preparedness. Nursing programs need plans to address the impact of extreme weather (e.g., food shortages, local fires, temporary program and/or clinical agency closures, other student impacts). These activities need to occur with a focus on the interest of key constituents, social justice, and cultural sensitivity.

### *Curriculum Integration*

Planetary health can be scaffolded throughout the curriculum, including incorporation into patient assessments and simulation experiences. Specific content can include the long-term implications of disasters and the impact of planetary health on disease prevalence and progression. Nursing programs also can consider developing a graduate specialty program focused on planetary health.

### *Faculty Development*

Faculty development is needed due to the influence of planetary health on nursing education. Faculty can learn about resource use and participate in focused discussions on planetary health and the curriculum. Faculty champions can be identified to lead school efforts.

### *Innovation and Change*

Faculty can develop innovations in teaching and learning activities to promote student learning in planetary health. For example, faculty can create a new board game on planetary health. Faculty also can innovate medical waste solutions. Nurses in general also can explore innovations for planetary health. To achieve innovations, funding needs to be provided to trial projects.

### *Challenges and Barriers*

A general numbness to planetary health can impede change. Discussants also reported that they perceive nurses have limited power to influence change. However, they also reported that the failure of nurses to address planetary health can ultimately affect their students' health. Faculty's lack of readiness, expertise, and capacity building further limits potential impact. The politically charged nature of the topic also limits civil conversation that could positively influence outcomes.

## CONCLUSION

Planetary health is generally identified as an important topic for nursing and nursing academia. However, there are mixed views on how to incorporate planetary health into nursing curricula, if at all. With curricula already overloaded and focused on acute-care nursing, embedding planetary health into curricula will be challenging. To make a positive impact, faculty need to commit to professional development, serve as champions, incorporate content into their courses, redesign curricula, and role model positive behaviors.

### *References*

Dogan, E. I. K., Ekiz, P., & Meyer, C. G. (2025). Planetary health education for nursing students: A scoping review. *Nurse Education Today, 153*, 106812. https://doi.org/10.1016/j.nedt.2025.106812

Levett-Jones, T., Catling, C., Cheer, S., Fields, L., Foster, A., Maguire, J., Mcintyre, E., Moroney, T., Pich, J., Pitt, V., Whiteing, N., & Lokmic-Tomkins, Z. (2025). Achieving consensus on the essential knowledge and skills needed by nursing students to promote planetary health and sustainable healthcare: A Delphi study. *Journal of Advanced Nursing, 81*, 8281–8299. https://doi.org/10.1111/jan.16229

Lokmic-Tomkins, Z., Schenk, E. C., Lee, J. L., & Moorley, C., (2025). Upholding planetary health through nursing leadership in a fragmented global landscape. *Journal of Advanced Nursing, 81*, 8063–8065. https://doi.org/10.1111/jan.70247

National League for Nursing Climate Change and Health Strategic Action Group. (2022, September). *NLN vision statement: Climate change and health*. National League for Nursing. https://www.nln.org/docs/default-source/default-document-library/vision-series-climate-change-health.pdf?sfvrsn=86ee3340_3

Vandenberg, S., Strus, J. A., Chircop, A., Egert, A., & Savard, J. (2025). Planetary health in nursing: A scoping review. *Journal of Advanced Nursing, 81*, 8080–8115. https://doi.org/10.1111/jan.16570

PART 5

# Nurse and Nursing Faculty Well-Being

# 10

# Overview of Nurse and Nursing Faculty Well-Being

**Cynda Hylton Rushton**

## NURSING WORKFORCE SHORTAGES WORLDWIDE

Global nursing shortages exacerbate stress and compromise patient care. Policy and planning barriers, limited training capacity, turnover, and burnout drive these shortages (Tamata & Mohammadnezhad, 2023). ICN (2021) underscores the urgency of addressing workforce recruitment and retention. According to the ICN's (2021) Global Nursing Shortage and Nurse Retention report, 90 percent of National Nurses Associations (NNAs) are somewhat or extremely concerned that heavy workloads, insufficient resourcing, and pandemic-related burnout are driving increased numbers of nurses to leave the profession and raising intentions to leave nursing postpandemic. Approximately 20 percent of NNAs reported an increase of nurses leaving in 2020, and studies worldwide consistently highlight elevated intention-to-leave rates. Nursing workforce shortage is a global challenge rooted in multiple causes, such as individual, educational, organizational and managerial, and policymaking factors (Tamata & Mohammadnezhad, 2023).

Given the existing nursing shortage, the aging workforce, and COVID-19's impact, ICN (2021) estimates that up to 13 million nurses will be needed globally to fill the gap. More than 70 percent of NNAs state that their countries plan to expand nursing school enrollment, yet they caution there will be a three- to four-year gap before these graduates can join the workforce—during which an exodus of experienced nurses is feared (ICN, 2021). Faculty shortages compound the problem, restricting the preparation of new nurses. In the United States alone, over 65,000 qualified applicants were denied admission to nursing programs in 2023 due to faculty and resource limitations (American Association of Colleges of Nursing [AACN], 2024). ICN calls on governments to act decisively now to mitigate turnover and strengthen nurse recruitment, retention, and well-being.

## NURSE WELL-BEING

Nurse well-being is vitally important to address the current nursing workforce challenges. Nurse well-being is a holistic state of physical, mental, emotional, and professional health that enables nurses to function effectively, feel fulfilled in their work, and remain resilient amid occupational stressors. It encompasses job satisfaction, psychological safety, physical health, work-life balance, and a sense of purpose and connection within health care environments. ICN (2021) defines nurse well-being as a dynamic, multidimensional construct influenced by personal resources, work environment, organizational culture, and professional identity.

## CURRENT STATE OF NURSE WELL-BEING

### Burnout and Mental Health

Globally, nurses report high levels of burnout driven by heavy workloads, emotional strain, and insufficient staffing—pressures intensified by the COVID-19 pandemic (Martin et al., 2023; Shah et al., 2021; Woo et al., 2020). Burnout prevalence varies widely, from about 11 percent overall (Woo et al., 2020) to over 80 percent in some sub-Saharan African settings (Owuor et al., 2020). Intensive care unit nurses experience particularly high rates, with a pooled prevalence of 44 percent and peaks of 61 percent during the pandemic (Papazian et al., 2023). Emergency department nurses report comparable levels (Alanazy & Alruwaili, 2023). Mental health challenges—including depression, anxiety, posttraumatic stress disorder, and suicidal ideation—are pervasive (d'Ettorre et al., 2021).

### Moral Suffering in Response to Ethical Challenges

Nurses often experience ethical conflict, especially in crises, leading to long-term emotional harm and moral suffering (Lake et al., 2022). The frequency of these is exacerbated during crises when they cannot act in alignment with ethical beliefs and values (Morley et al., 2020). In response to them, moral suffering ensues, manifesting as moral distress or moral injury (Rushton, 2023). Scarcity of resources and institutional constraints, such as visitation policies, were associated with higher degrees of moral suffering and elevated mental health outcomes in nurses (Kok et al., 2021; McMillan et al., 2021; Smallwood et al., 2021; Stein et al., 2021). These patterns also were evident in nurse leaders (Bergman et al., 2025). The contribution of moral suffering to degraded well-being is a frequently overlooked factor and important consideration when designing interventions to support nurse well-being and integrity.

### Organizational Factors

Lack of leadership support, poor workplace culture, limited autonomy, and insufficient recognition worsen well-being (Kohnen et al., 2024). Long shifts, irregular schedules, and limited recovery time lead to chronic fatigue and poor work–life balance (Farag et al., 2022; Zhang et al., 2020), which can be magnified in countries where resource constraints and systemic understaffing intensify stress and burnout. Similar patterns are recognized in nursing faculty (Dugger, 2024). Organizational factors also are associated with symptoms of moral injury and degraded well-being outcomes (Scoglio et al., 2024).

## Contributing Factors to Well-Being

A growing evidence base highlights modifiable organizational and individual factors that support nurse well-being. Positive work environments with strong leadership, collegial support, and effective communication improve outcomes (Gebreheat et al., 2023). Adequate nursing resources reduce stress and prevent burnout (Li et al., 2024). Psychological safety, resilience training, and access to mental health resources promote job satisfaction and retention (Foster et al., 2019). Flexible scheduling, supportive leave policies, and recognition of professional contributions further enhance well-being (Boamah et al., 2023; Han., 2023; Kohnen et al., 2024). The absence of these factors contributes to degraded nurse well-being.

## Nursing Faculty Well-Being

Nursing faculty face similar risks of burnout and diminished well-being with predictors including heavy workload, salary constraints, and work-life imbalance (Dugger, 2024). Faculty report pressures to maintain clinical competence, meet research expectations, and manage high student-faculty ratios, all within cultures that may tolerate incivility or toxic leadership (Aldhafeeri & Alanazi, 2024). Faculty shortages disrupt student learning, hinder clinical preparation, and threaten institutional reputation (Anderson et al., 2024; Antig et al., 2024). Beyond this, learning from faculty who are exhausted or burned out can expose new nurses to role models who undermine sustainability in the profession (D'Aoust et al., 2024).

## Resilience as a Protective Resource

Researchers consistently report a moderate to large inverse relationship between resilience and burnout among health care professionals, lower turnover intention, and higher work engagement (Castillo-González et al., 2024; Nantsupawat et al., 2024). For nursing faculty, resilience supports well-being by strengthening coping skills, promoting a balanced stress appraisal, enriching social connections, and improving work-life integration. Rothacker-Peyton et al. (2022) found that nursing faculty had average resilience scores comparable to the U.S. population, although a higher percentage of nursing faculty were on the lower spectrum for resilience. Singh et al. (2020) likewise identified resilience as a protective factor, reinforced by collegial relationships, positive outlooks, and reflective practice. Similarly, moral resilience, a distinct type of resilience, has been shown to be a protective resource for nurses and nurse leaders (Rushton, 2023).

While some critics have dismissed investing in resilience as merely enabling individuals to tolerate unacceptable systemic conditions (Traynor, 2024), this perspective fundamentally misunderstands the true nature of resilience. Genuine resilience is not the passive acceptance of injustice and hardship, but rather an active process of recognizing one's circumstances clearly and choosing to transcend them. This capacity to harness our inherent resilient potential has served as the foundation for human survival and progress throughout history.

As Frankl (1946/2006) powerfully asserted: "Everything can be taken from a man but one thing: the last of the human freedoms—to choose one's attitude in any given set of circumstances, to choose one's own way. When we are no longer able to change a situation, we are challenged to change ourselves" (p. 66). While comprehensive attention must certainly be given to the systemic factors within the nursing ecosystem that impact well-being, dismissing resilience as a protective resource that can be cultivated and amplified risks abandoning a vital human capacity that remains within everyone's control. Rather than perpetuating oppression, developing resilience can restore agency and professional integrity, empowering nurses to navigate challenges while advocating for necessary systemic change.

## EVIDENCE-INFORMED STRATEGIES TO IMPROVE NURSE WELL-BEING

A growing perspective suggests that interventions are needed at both the individual and system levels to create the conditions for nurses to thrive (AACN, 2020; NASEM, 2019; NLN, 2021). Consistent with polarity management, an overemphasis on either aspect of the equation can create imbalance and result in unintended consequences (Johnson, 2014). Focusing exclusively on individual strategies can create undue pressure on nurses to be overly responsible for their well-being and relieve health care systems of the responsibility for creating healthy workplaces. Similarly, focusing solely on the system or organization does not account for the interrelated aspects of our human experience and can divert attention from empowering individuals to invest in their own self-stewardship (Rushton, 2024). Although there are significant structural contributors to nurse well-being, there is shared responsibility between nurses and their clinical practice and academic environments.

There are a variety of promising evidence informed strategies for fostering nurse well-being. Table 10.1 outlines selected strategies that offer promising interventions to expand nurses' repertoire of skills and tools to meet the complexity of health care and academic realities. Skills such as mindfulness, meditation, and self-compassion build the necessary neuropathways to support stability amid challenges. Sleep and physical activity support physiologic and functional health while cognitive behavioral therapy, journaling, gratitude practices, art, and music support psychological well-being. Importantly, group activities support connection and reduce isolation. While not an exhaustive list, these interventions and others offer a promising direction to support individual nurse well-being.

These approaches, when combined with organizational interventions, offer the strongest protection against burnout and mental distress. Organizational resources are critical to nurse well-being and burnout prevention, extending beyond individual factors. Informal resources—such as supportive social relationships and positive organizational norms—bolster well-being through psychological mechanisms like perceived organizational support, psychological safety, and social identity. Consistent with social cognitive theory (Bandura, 2001), which highlights the influence of environment on behavior and health, these resources can either buffer or intensify the effects of job demands in academic settings. Nursing programs with strong organizational climates—characterized by high recognition, psychological safety, and work-life support—show significantly lower faculty turnover intentions, with workplace culture and work-life balance emerging as the strongest predictors of faculty retention and career satisfaction (Boamah et al., 2023).

**TABLE 10.1**

**Selected Evidence-Informed Individual Interventions for Nurse and Nursing Faculty Well-Being**

| Intervention | Description |
|---|---|
| Mindfulness and Meditation (Hsu et al., 2024; Karakurt et al., 2025; Wang et al., 2023) | Reduces stress and emotional exhaustion; improves focus and emotional regulation. |
| Self-Compassion Training (Bian et al., 2025) | Builds emotional resilience; reduces self-criticism and burnout. |
| Physical Activity (Hsu et al., 2024) | Enhances mood and sleep quality; reduces stress and anxiety. |
| Sleep Hygiene (Malewska et al., 2025; Membrive-Jiménez et al., 2022) | Supports cognitive recovery; reduces burnout. |
| Cognitive Behavioral Therapy (Badriyah et al., 2025) | Helps manage anxiety, depression, and stress through cognitive restructuring. |
| Journaling and Gratitude Practice (Cochran & Mealer., 2023) | Promotes optimism and emotional processing; reduces stress. |
| Digital Resilience Training (Yu et al., 2024) | Online tools improve resilience and emotional regulation. |
| Peer Support and Group Work (Loo et al., 2022) | Strengthens social connection; reduces isolation; increases psychological safety. |

A German study revealed that health care resilience during COVID-19 involves cross-level interdependence, where individual resilience and organizational resilience work together rather than independently, with organizational resilience serving as a critical mediator that enhances individual adaptation and team efficacy, ultimately leading to more positive perceptions of pandemic-related transformation across all levels of the health care system (Gröschke et al., 2022). Table 10.2 offers selected system-focused interventions that may affect nurses practicing in all settings.

## The Total Worker Framework

The National Institute for Occupational Safety and Health's (2024) Total Worker Health approach recognizes that work is a powerful social determinant of health and calls for interventions that strengthen both individual and organizational factors, an especially urgent priority in nursing. Research shows that targeting only personal resilience or only system change yields limited results, while combining them may amplify the benefits. A national study of 2,004 Veterans Administration health care workers found that moral injury risk was strongly predicted by modifiable organizational factors including perceived lack of management support for worker health and safety, supervisor support, coworker support, and empowerment to make job-related decisions, demonstrating clear alignment with Total Worker Health principles that integrate individual well-being with organizational culture and workplace conditions to comprehensively address worker health outcomes (Purcell et al., 2024). For nursing faculty, effective programs may combine resilience training with recognition initiatives, physical activity with psychological safety efforts, or sleep education with improvements in work-family culture. Adopting a multi-level approach acknowledges the complex, interdependent factors that influence faculty well-being. This perspective aligns with the Total Worker Health framework, which integrates individual and organizational strategies to prevent burnout and promote sustained professional fulfillment. Ongoing research led by D'Aoust and colleagues is further examining how such combined interventions enhance resilience, engagement, and retention within academic nursing environments. The $R^3$: Resilient Nurses' Initiative exemplifies this integrated model (Rushton et al., 2025), demonstrating early evidence of improved well-being, a strengthened organizational climate, and reduced turnover intentions.

**TABLE 10.2**

**Selected Evidence-Informed Systemic Interventions for Nurse and Nursing Faculty Well-Being**

| Intervention | Description |
|---|---|
| Leadership and Managerial Support (Alsadaan et al., 2023) | Supportive, visible, and communicative leadership is linked to improved morale, lower stress, and reduced burnout in nurses. |
| Flexible Scheduling and Workload Management (Aust et al., 2024) | Adequate staffing and manageable workloads reduce fatigue and prevent burnout. Flexible scheduling improves work-life balance. |
| Resilience and Wellness Programs (Dzau et al., 2024; Melnyk et al., 2022) | Institution-led resilience training and wellness workshops can decrease stress and improve emotional regulation and retention. |
| Mental Health Access Services (Doran, 2022; Hindman et al., 2024; Ilola et al., 2024) | Onsite or digital access to psychological services improves coping and reduces mental health symptoms in nurses. |
| Shared Governance and Inclusion (NASEM, 2021) | Giving nurses a voice in decision-making improves engagement, job satisfaction, and a sense of control. |
| Safe and Supportive Work Environments (Guerriero et al., 2025; NASEM, 2021) | Addressing incivility, violence, and moral distress contributes to psychological safety and team cohesion. |
| Recognition and Incentive Programs (Sweeney, 2021; Wocial et al., 2023) | Acknowledging and rewarding nurse contributions fosters motivation, morale, and retention. |
| Healthy Physical Work Environment (Krishnanmoorthy et al., 2025) | Ergonomic tools, safe staffing ratios, rest breaks, and calm spaces improve physical and psychological well-being. |

## The Way Forward

Improving nurse and nursing faculty well-being requires a multimodal approach grounded in a social ecological framework that acknowledges the interconnection and synergy among all aspects of the ecosystem where nurses practice (Davidson et al., 2018) (see Figure 10.1). Regardless of whether nurses are in clinical practice or academia, attention must be given to how interventions in any dimension impact others to avoid unintended consequences. Engaging in a comprehensive approach to amplify individual capacities and resilience while dismantling the systemic contributors is likely to produce the most sustainable results. Frameworks such as U.S. Surgeon General's (2022) Five Essentials for Workplace Mental Health and Well-Being, NASEM's (2021) System Approach, American Association of Critical-care Nurses (2016) Healthy Work Environment Standards, and others provide useful starting points to guide design and implementation.

For academia, NASEM (2019) recommended cultivating positive learning environments by:

1. Implementing programs that support faculty and learner well-being.
2. Investing in leadership roles dedicated to well-being.
3. Aligning incentives and reward structures to model and foster well-being.
4. Creating broad systems of support and routinely assessing well-being with validated measures.
5. Monitoring and adjusting workloads while removing barriers to accessing resources and reducing stigma.

The NASEM (2019) recommendations, in conjunction with the policy directives outlined in the *Future of Nursing 2020–2030* report (NASEM, 2021), underscore the critical role of educational institutions in fortifying nursing education with a focus on well-being

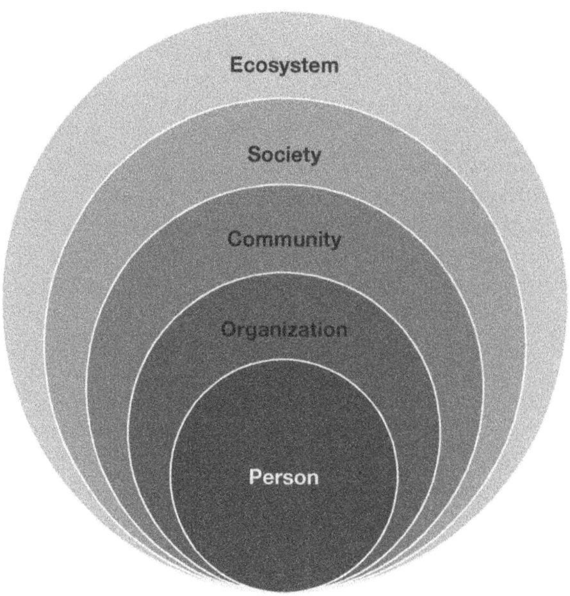


**FIGURE 10.1:** Social Ecological Framework (Source: Davidson et al., 2018).

and resilience. These recommendations were further validated by NCSBN (2021), whose endorsement is reflected in the updated *The Essentials: Core Competencies for Professional Nursing Education* (AACN, 2021). This revision highlights personal health, resilience, and well-being as integral components of Domain 10: Personal, Professional, and Leadership Development, positioning them as fundamental pillars for the holistic preparation of future nurses.

## CONCLUSION

Nurse and nursing faculty well-being is essential to sustaining the global workforce, delivering high-quality patient care, and preparing future generations of nurses. Evidence shows that combining organizational reforms with individualized resilience strategies reduces burnout, strengthens retention, and enhances professional fulfillment. Healthy faculty create learning environments that model well-being, foster psychological safety and inclusion, and promote positive outcomes for students and colleagues. Achieving this requires sustained investment in systemic change across the health care ecosystem and a broad set of resources to meet the complexity and demands of today's nursing workforce. Thus, a multimodal approach to improve and retain the nursing workforce requires strategies to enhance social, emotional, and moral resilience; well-being; and ethical practice in nursing with concerted efforts to transform the culture of health systems and professional education.

### References

Alanazy, A. R. M., & Alruwaili, A. (2023). The global prevalence and associated factors of burnout among emergency department healthcare workers and the impact of the COVID-19 pandemic: A systematic review and meta-analysis. *Healthcare*, *11*(15), 2220. https://doi.org/10.3390/healthcare11152220

Aldhafeeri, N. A., & Alanazi, F. J. (2024). Intent to leave academia: Perceptions and challenges of nurse faculty. *BMC Nursing, 23,* 506. https://doi.org/10.1186/s12912-024-02137-y

Alsadaan, N., Salameh, B., Reshia, F. A. A. E., Alruwaili, R. F., Alruwaili, M., Ali, S. A. A., Alruwaili, A. N., Hefnawy, G. R., Alshammari, M. S. S., Alrumayh, A. G. R., Alruwaili, A. O., & Jones, L. K. (2023). Impact of nurse leaders behaviors on nursing staff performance: A systematic review of literature. *Inquiry, 60*, 1–14. https://doi.org/10.3390/admsci13060142

American Association of Colleges of Nursing. (2020, August). *A call to action for academic nurse leaders to promote practices to enhance optimal well-being, resilience, and suicide prevention in schools of nursing across the U.S.* American Association of Colleges of Nursing. https://www.aacnnursing.org/portals/0/pdfs/position-statements/7-2020-Resolution-For-AACN-Nurse-Wellness-Suicide-Prevention.pdf

American Association of Colleges of Nursing. (2021). *The essentials: Core competencies for professional nursing education.* American Association of Colleges of Nursing. https://www.aacnnursing.org/Portals/0/PDFs/Publications/Essentials-2021.pdf

American Association of Colleges of Nursing. (2024). *2023–2024 enrollment and graduations in baccalaureate and graduate programs in nursing.* American Association of Colleges of Nursing.

American Association of Critical-care Nurses. (2016). *AACN standards for establishing and sustaining healthy work environments: A journey to excellence* (2nd ed.). American Association of Critical-care Nurses. https://www.aacn.org/nursing-excellence/

standards/aacn-standards-for-establishing-and-sustaining-healthy-work-environments

Anderson, M., Taylor, N., Rowley, T., Owens, C., & Iacob, E. (2024). Understanding factors influencing nursing faculty departure and intentions. *Nurse Educator, 49*(4), 222–226. https://doi.org/10.1097/NNE.0000000000001612

Antig, A., Arañez, S., Cañazares, C., & Palompon, D. (2024). Nursing faculty shortage impact on nursing students: A descriptive phenomenological study. *Nursing Research and Practice, 2024,* 1751942. https://doi.org/10.1155/2024/1751942

Aust, B., Leduc, C., Cresswell-Smith, J., O'Brien, C., Rugulies, R., Leduc, M., Dhalaigh, D. N., Dushaj, A., Fanaj, N., Guinart, D., Maxwell, M., Reich, H., Ross, V., Sadath, A., Schnitzspahn, K., Tóth, M. D., van Audenhove, C., van Weeghel, J., Wahlbeck, K., Arensman, E., & Greiner, B. A. (2024). The effects of different types of organizational workplace mental health interventions on mental health and wellbeing in healthcare workers: A systematic review. *International Archives of Occupational and Environmental Health, 97*(4), 485–522. https://doi.org/10.1007/s00420-024-02065-z

Badriyah, F. L., Suarilah, I., Tarihoran, E. T. A. U., Saragih, I. D., & Lee, B. (2025). Effectiveness of cognitive behavioral therapy in reducing psychological distress in nurses: A systematic review and meta-analysis of experimental studies. *Nursing & Health Sciences, 27*(1), e70036. https://doi.org/10.1111/nhs.70036

Bandura, A. (2001). Social cognitive theory: An agentic perspective. *Annual Review of Psychology, 52*, 1–26. https://doi.org/10.1146/annurev.psych.52.1.1

Bergman, A. J.., Hanson, G. C., Jenkins, C., Nelson, K., Boyce, D., & Rushton, C. H. (2025) Moral injury, moral resilience, and organizational effectiveness among nurse leaders: A descriptive analysis during the COVID-19 pandemic. *BMC Nursing, 24*(1), 1100. https://doi.org/10.1186/s12912-025-03744-z

Bian, J., Chen, F., Fang, S., & Wang, Y. (2025). Self-compassion intervention programs for nurses: A scoping review. *Healthcare, 13*, 177. https://doi.org/10.3390/healthcare13020177

Boamah, S. A., Kalu, M. E., Havaei, F., McMillan, K., & Belita, E. (2023). Predictors of nursing faculty job and career satisfaction, turnover intentions, and professional outlook: A national survey. *Healthcare, 11*(14), 2099. https://doi.org/10.3390/healthcare11142099

Castillo-González, A., Velando-Soriano, A., De La Fuente-Solana, E. I., Martos-Cabrera, B. M., Membrive-Jiménez, M. J., Ramírez-Baena, L., & Cañadas-De La Fuente, G. A. (2024). Relation and effect of resilience on burnout in nurses: A literature review and meta-analysis. *International Nursing Review, 71*(1), 160–167. https://doi.org/10.1111/inr.12838

Cochran, K. L., & Mealer, M. (2023). An evaluation of a narrative expressive writing program for nurses during the COVID-19 pandemic. *The Journal of Nursing Administration, 53*(4), 228–233. https://doi.org/10.1097/NNA.0000000000001274

D'Aoust, R., Sarver, L., Swoboda, S. Hughes, R. Hudson, K., Wright, E., & Rushton, C. (2024). An integrative review of burnout and related concepts in nursing faculty. *Journal of Nursing Education and Practice, 14*(1), 1–11. https://doi.org/10.5430/jnep.v14n1p1

Davidson, P., Rushton, C. H., Kurtz, M., Wise, B., Jackson, D., Beaman, A., & Broome, M. (2018). A social-ecological framework: A model for addressing ethical practice in nursing. *Journal of Clinical Nursing, 27*(5-6), e1233–e1241. https://doi.org/10.1111/jocn.14158

d'Ettorre, G., Ceccarelli, G., Santinelli, L., Vassalini, P., Innocenti, G. P., Alessandri, F., Koukopoulos, A. E., Russo, A., d'Ettorre, G., & Tarsitani, L. (2021). Post-traumatic stress symptoms in healthcare workers dealing with the COVID-19 pandemic: A systematic review. *International Journal of Environmental Research and Public Health, 18*(2), 601. https://doi.org/10.3390/ijerph18020601

Doran, M. (2022). Employee assistance programs: A misunderstood and underused resource for nurses. *Journal of Nursing Administration, 52*(11), 625-627. https://doi.org/10.1097/nna.0000000000001200

Dugger, J. (2024). Predictive and associated factors of burnout in nursing faculty:

An integrative review. *Nurse Educator, 49*(3), E142–E146. https://doi.org/10.1097/NNE.0000000000001533

Farag, A., Scott, L., Perkhounkova, Y., Saeidzadeh, S., & Hein, M. (2022). Human factors approach to evaluate predictors of acute care nurse occupational fatigue. *Applied Ergonomics, 100*, 103647. https://doi.org/10.1016/j.apergo.2021.103647

Foster, K., Roche, M., Delgado, C., Cuzzillo, C., Giandinoto, J. A., & Furness, T. (2019). Resilience and mental health nursing: An integrative review of international literature. *International Journal of Mental Health Nursing, 28*(1), 71–85. https://doi.org/10.1111/inm.12548

Frankl, V. E. (1946/2006). *Man's search for meaning* (I. Lasch, Trans.; 4th ed.). Beacon Press.

Gebreheat, G., Teame, H., & Costa, E. I. (2023). The impact of transformational leadership style on nurses' job satisfaction: An integrative review. *SAGE Open Nursing, 9*, 23779608231197428. https://doi.org/10.1177/23779608231197428

Gröschke, D., Hofmann, E., Müller, N. D., & Wolf, J. (2022). Individual and organizational resilience—Insights from healthcare providers in Germany during the COVID-19 pandemic. *Frontiers in Psychology, 13*, 965380. https://doi.org/10.3389/fpsyg.2022.965380

Han, S. (2023). Nurses' job crafting, work engagement, and well-being: A path analysis. *BMC Nursing, 22*, 405. https://doi.org/10.1186/s12912-023-01573-6

Hindman, J., Zugai, J., & Raeburn, T. (2024). Digital applications potential to support the mental well-being of nurses: An integrative review. *Mental Health and Digital Technologies, 1*(2), 212–227. https://doi.org/10.1108/MHDT-12-2023-0006

Hsu, H., Lee, H., Hung, H., Chen, Y., Yen, M., Chiang, H., Chow, L., Fetzer, S. J., & Mu, P. (2024). Effectiveness of individual-based strategies to reduce nurse burnout: An umbrella review. *Journal of Nursing Management, 2024*(1), 8544725. https://doi.org/10.1155/2024/8544725

Ilola, T., Malmisalo, M., Laukka, E., Lehtiniemi, H., Pölkki, T., Kääriäinen, M., He, H.-G., & Kanste, O. (2024). The effectiveness of digital solutions in improving nurses' and healthcare professionals' mental well-being: A systematic review and meta-analysis. *Journal of Research in Nursing, 29*(2), 97–109. https://doi.org/10.1177/17449871241226914

International Council of Nurses. (2021, March 11). *ICN policy brief – The global nursing shortage and nurse retention.* International Council of Nurses. https://www.icn.ch/node/1297

Johnson, B. (2014). *Polarity management: Identifying and managing unsolvable problems*. HRS Press.

Karakurt, N., & Durmaz, H. (2025). The impact of mindfulness intervention on the subjective well-being of nursing students: An experimental study. *BMC Psychology, 13*, 955. https://doi.org/10.1186/s40359-025-03334-3

Kohnen, D., De Witte, H., Schaufeli, W. B., Dello, S., Bruyneel, L., & Sermeus, W. (2024). Engaging leadership and nurse well-being: The role of the work environment and work motivation—A cross-sectional study. *Human Resources for Health, 22*, 48. https://doi.org/10.1186/s12960-023-00886-6

Kok, N., van Gurp, J., Teerenstra, S., van der Hoeven, J. G., & Zegers, M. (2021). Complex interplay between moral distress and other risk factors of burnout in ICU professionals: Findings from a cross-sectional survey study. *BMJ Quality & Safety, 32*(4), 225–234. https://doi.org/10.1136/bmjqs-2020-012239

Krishnanmoorthy, G., Rampal, S., Karuthan, S. R., Baharudin, F., & Krishna, R. (2025). Effectiveness of participatory ergonomic interventions on work-related musculoskeletal disorders, sick absenteeism, and work performance among nurses: Systematic review. *JMIR Human Factors, 12*(1), e68522. https://doi.org/10.2196/68522

Lake, E. T., Narva, A. M., Holland, S., Smith, J. G., Cramer, E., Rosenbaum, K. E. F., French, R., Clark, R. R. S., & Rogowski, J. A. (2022). Hospital nurses' moral distress and mental health during COVID-19. *Journal of Advanced Nursing, 78*(3), 799–809. https://doi.org/10.1111/jan.15013

Lama, A., Nwamu, H., & Kim, Y. (2025). Interventions to address clinical incivility in nursing: A systematic review. *Nursing Reports, 15*(6), 199. https://doi.org/10.3390/nursrep15060199

Li, L. Z., Yang, P., & Singer, S. J. (2024). Nurse burnout and patient safety, satisfaction, and quality of care: A systematic review and meta-analysis. *JAMA Network Open, 7*(11), e2443059. https://doi.org/10.1001/jamanetworkopen.2024.43059

Loo, J. H., Bone, L., Forte, J., Kirley, E., Lynch T., & Aboumatar, H. (2022). The benefits and challenges of established peer support programmes for patients, informal caregivers, and healthcare providers. *Family Practice, 39*, 903–912. https://doi.org/10.1093/fampra/cmac004

Malewska, K., Serafin, L., & Czarkowska-Paczek, B. (2025). The relationship between sleep quality and resilience among intensive care unit nurses: A cross-sectional study. *Nursing in Critical Care, 30*(2), e70010. https://doi.org/10.1111/nicc.70010

Martin, B., Kaminski-Ozturk, N., O'Hara, C., & Smiley, R. (2023). Examining the impact of the COVID-19 pandemic on burnout and stress among U.S. nurses. *Journal of Nursing Regulation*, *14*(1), 4–12. https://doi.org/10.1016/S2155-8256(23)00063-7

McMillan, K., Wright, D. K., McPherson, C. J., Ma, K., & Bitzas, V. (2021). Visitor restrictions, palliative care, and epistemic agency: A qualitative study of nurses' relational practice during the coronavirus pandemic. *Global Qualitative Nursing Research*, *8*, 1–12. https://doi.org/10.1177/23333936211051702

Melnyk, B. M., Hsieh, A. P., Tan, A., Teall, A., Weberg, D., Jun, J., Gawlik, K., & Hoying, H. (2022). Associations among nurses' mental/physical health, lifestyle behaviors, shift length, and workplace wellness support during COVID-19: Important implications for health care systems. *Nursing Administration Quarterly, 46*(1), 5–18. https://doi.org/10.1097/NAQ.0000000000000499

Membrive-Jiménez, M. J., Gómez-Urquiza, J. L., Suleiman-Martos, N., Velando-Soriano, A., Ariza, T., De la Fuente-Solana, E. I., & Cañadas-De la Fuente, G. A. (2022). Relation between Burnout and Sleep Problems in Nurses: A Systematic Review with Meta-Analysis. *Healthcare, 10*(5), 954. https://doi.org/10.3390/healthcare10050954

Morley, G., Grady, C., McCarthy, J., & Ulrich, C. M. (2020). COVID-19: Ethical challenges for nurses. *Hastings Center Report, 50*(3), 35–39. https://doi.org/10.1002/hast.1110

Nantsupawat, A., Kutney-Lee, A., Abhichart-tibutra, K., Wichaikhum, O.-A., & Poghosyan, L. (2024). Exploring the relationships between resilience, burnout, work engagement, and intention to leave among nurses in the context of the COVID-19 pandemic: A cross-sectional study. *BMC Nursing, 23*, 290. https://doi.org/10.1186/s12912-024-01958-1

National Academies of Sciences, Engineering, and Medicine. (2019). Taking action against clinician burnout: A systems approach to professional well-being. *The National Academies Press*. https://doi.org/10.17226/25521

National Academies of Sciences, Engineering, and Medicine. (2021). *The future of nursing 2020–2030: Charting a path to achieve health equity. The National Academies Press*. https://doi.org/10.17226/25982

National Council of State Boards of Nursing. (2021). *The future of nursing report, 2020–2023: Charting a path to achieve health equity [Policy briefing*]. National Council of State Boards of Nursing. https://www.ncsbn.org/news/the-future-of-nursing-report-2020-2030

National Institute for Occupational Safety and Health. (2024, May 31). *About the Total Worker Health® approach [Internet*]. National Institute for Occupational Safety and Health. https://www.cdc.gov/niosh/twh/about/index.html

National League for Nursing. (2021). *NLN value statement on workforce demands of the future: The educational imperative.* National League for Nursing. https://www.nln.org/detail-pages/news/2021/11/09/nln-value-statement-on-workforce-demands-of-the-future-the-educational-imperative

Owuor, R. A., Mutungi, K., Anyango, R., & Mwita, C. C. (2020). Prevalence of burnout among nurses in sub-Saharan Africa: a systematic review. *JBI Evidence Synthesis, 18*(6), 1189–1207. https://doi.org/10.11124/JBISRIR-D-19-00170

Papazian, L., Hraiech, S., Loundou, A., Herridge, M. S., Boyer, L., et al. (2023). High-level burnout in physicians and nurses working in adult ICUs: A systematic review and meta-analysis. *Intensive Care Medicine, 49*, 387–400. https://doi.org/10.1007/s00134-023-07025-8

Purcell, N., Bertenthal, D., Usman, H., Griffin, B. J., Maguen, S., McGrath, S., Smith, M. W., Sato, K., Thomas, E., & Hysong, S. J. (2024). Moral injury and mental health in healthcare workers are linked to organizational culture and modifiable workplace conditions: Results of a national, mixed-methods study conducted at Veterans Affairs (VA) medical centers during the COVID-19 pandemic. *PLOS Mental Health, 1*(7), e0000085. https://doi.org/10.1371/journal.pmen.0000085

Rothacker-Peyton S., Wilson-Anderson K., & Mayer K. (2022) Nursing faculty professional quality of life and resilience in a changing educational environment. *Journal of Nursing Education, 61*(6):330–333. https://doi.org/10.3928/01484834-20220404-12

Rushton, C. H. (2023) Transforming moral suffering by cultivating moral resilience and ethical practice. *American Journal of Critical Care, 32*(4), 238–248. https://doi.org/10.4037/ajcc2023207

Rushton, C. H. (2024). Self-stewardship: An ethical imperative for nurses. *AACN Advanced Critical Care, 35*(2), 193–198. https://doi.org/10.4037/aacnacc2024727

Rushton, C. H., Swoboda, S., Reller, N., Sarver, L., Wright, E., Hudson, K., Hughes, V., Hanson, G., & D'Aoust, R. (2025) Conceptual model and design of an initiative to build nurses' resilience and ethical practice. *Journal of Professional Nursing, 61*(6), 33–40. https://doi.org/10.1016/j.profnurs.2025.08.008

Scoglio, A. A. J., Stelson, E. A., Becene, I., Marquez, C. I., & Rich-Edwards, J. W. (2024). A mixed methods analysis of moral injury among healthcare workers during the COVID-19 pandemic. *PLOS One, 19*(7), e0304620. https://doi.org/10.1371/journal.pone.0304620

Shah, M. K., Gandrakota, N., & Cimiotto, J. P. (2021). Prevalence of and factors associated with nurse burnout in the US. *JAMA Network Open, 4*(2), e2036469. https://doi.org/10.1001/jamanetworkopen.2020.36469

Singh, C., Cross, W., Munro, I., & Jackson, D. (2020). Occupational stress facing nurse academics-a mixed-methods systematic review. *Journal of Clinical Nursing, 29*(5-6), 720–735. https://doi.org/10.1111/jocn.15150

Smallwood, N., Pascoe, A., Karimi, L., & Willis, K. (2021). Moral distress and perceived community views are associated with mental health symptoms in frontline health workers during the COVID-19 pandemic. *International Journal of Environmental Research and Public Health, 18*(16), 8723. https://doi.org/10.3390/ijerph18168723

Stein, M. B., McGlinchey, R. E., & Patrick, S. W. (2021). Moral distress in frontline healthcare workers in the initial epicenter of the COVID-19 pandemic in the United States: Relationship to PTSD symptoms, burnout, and psychosocial functioning. *Depression and Anxiety, 38*(10), 1007–1017. https://doi.org/10.1002/da.23205

Sweeney, C. D. (2021). The value of recognition: The DAISY award. *Nursing Administration Quarterly, 45*(3), 253–261. https://doi.org/10.1097/naq.0000000000000478

Tamata, A. T., & Mohammadnezhad, M. (2023). A systematic review study on the factors affecting shortage of nursing workforce in the hospitals. *Nursing Open, 10*(3), 1247–1257. https://doi.org/10.1002/nop2.1434

Traynor, M. (2024). *Nursing, COVID and the end of resilience: A critical approach*. Routledge.

U.S. Surgeon General. (2022). *The U.S. Surgeon General's framework for workplace mental health & well-being*. U.S. Department of Health and Human Services. https://www.hhs.gov/sites/default/files/workplace-mental-health-well-being.pdf

Wang, Q., Wang, F., Zhang, S., Liu, C., Feng, Y., & Chen, J. (2023). Effects of a mindfulness-based interventions on stress, burnout in nurses: A systematic review and meta-analysis. *Frontiers in Psychology, 14*, 1218340. https://doi.org/10.3389/fpsyt.2023.1218340

Wocial, L. D., Miller, G., Montz, K., LaPradd, M., & Slaven, J. E. (2023). Evaluation of interventions to address moral distress: A multi-method approach. *HEC Forum, 36*, 373–401. https://doi.org/10.1007/s10730-023-09508-z

Woo, T., Ho, R. C., Tang, A., & Tam, W. W. S. (2020). Global prevalence of burnout symptoms among nurses: A systematic review and meta-analysis. *Journal of Psychiatric Research, 123*, 9–20. https://doi.org/10.1016/j.jpsychires.2019.12.015

Yu, F., Chu, G., Yeh, T., & Fernandez, R. (2024). Effects of interventions to promote resilience in nurses: A systematic review. *International Journal of Nursing Studies, 157*, 104825. https://doi.org/10.1016/j.ijnurstu.2024.104825

Zhang, Y., Wang, C., Pan, W., Zheng, J., Gao, J., Huang, X., Cai, S., Zhai, Y., Latour, J. M., & Zhu, C. (2020). Stress, burnout, and coping strategies of frontline nurses during the COVID-19 epidemic in Wuhan and Shanghai, China. *Frontiers in Psychiatry, 11*, 565520. https://doi.org/10.3389/fpsyt.2020.565520

# 11

# Barriers and Strategies for Incorporating Nurse and Nursing Faculty Well-Being Into Nursing Education

**Gordon Lee Gillespie and Sandra Davis**

## INTRODUCTION

Since the onset of the COVID-19 pandemic in 2020, nurse and nursing faculty well-being has worsened (Grubaugh et al., 2023). Interventions are needed to address this evolving problem for the workforce. Well-being initiatives need to be intentional and have leadership support (NLN Civil and Healthy Academic Work Environment SAG, 2018; Zangaro et al., 2025). Black et al. (2025) conducted a scoping review of the literature and identified several interventions to promote well-being in nursing education. For example, a wellness committee could be launched to oversee well-being efforts focusing on physical activity (e.g., walking groups, Zumba classes), social connections (e.g., eating lunch together, faculty debriefing at the end of a semester), mindfulness, and yoga (Black et al., 2025). Well-being also was incorporated into curricula: standalone courses, wellness presentations at student orientation, guest lectures in required courses, and mindfulness, resilience, reflection, and caring training (Black et al., 2025; Brodie, 2026; Snow et al., 2024). Well-being for nurses, particularly newly licensed nurses, can be improved by incorporating apps and other media for digital reflective practice, where nurses document their reflections about their well-being throughout the day (Bembridge et al., 2025). This reflexive practice has been shown to create a sense of community and opportunities for collaborative learning (Bembridge et al., 2025). Well-being is a modifiable characteristic that requires commitment and engagement from nurses, nursing faculty, and leadership.

## WORLD CAFÉ QUESTIONS

Following a presentation on nurse and nursing faculty well-being, Utstein attendees responded to one of three questions at their various tables. After predetermined periods of time, they rotated to different tables, allowing them to ultimately respond to all three questions. The three questions were:

1. What is nurse well-being?
2. What are the barriers to nurse well-being?
3. What are proposed solutions to creating sustainable healthy work environments where students, nurses, and nurse educators can thrive?

This chapter describes the findings based on discussants' responses to the three questions on nurse and nursing faculty well-being. Details on the data collection procedures are described in Chapter 2.

## FINDINGS

### Nurse and Nursing Faculty Well-Being

There are six themes that describe nurse and nursing faculty well-being. The themes are Holistic Health and Wellness, Professional Fulfillment and Meaning, Work-Life Harmony, Supportive Systems and Culture, Personal Growth and Self-Awareness, and Positive Outcomes and Broader Impact.

#### *Holistic Health and Wellness*

Nurse and nursing faculty well-being is represented by a mind-body-spirit wellness. It also represents physical, psychological, and emotional health, which leads to human flourishing. Well-being is characterized by balance, inner strength and resilience, and psychosocial physical mental integrity while feeling safe and healthy. Well-being is promoted by belonging, love, and a positive mind and body connection. Of note, though, well-being fluctuates and is not static.

### *Professional Fulfillment and Meaning*

Meaningful work and enjoying and/or loving an individual's profession can lead to professional satisfaction. Professional fulfillment and meaning vary by individual (e.g., differing perceptions of health, happiness, and joy). Well-being in this capacity is enhanced by autonomy, independence, and full engagement in the workplace. Lack of burnout, ability to do one's life's calling, and sense of doing meaningful things further contribute to professional fulfillment and meaning.

### *Work-Life Harmony*

Work-Life balance is represented by professional satisfaction, alignment between being and doing, and being able to smile at the end of the workday. Harmony is actualized between a sense of purpose and the ability to achieve one's purpose, which also can be described as work-life effectiveness. Strategies to promote work-life harmony include setting work boundaries, finding balance between work and personal life, working a shortened work week (e.g., four-day workweek), and managing competing life roles (e.g., work, life, family, etc.).

### *Supportive Systems and Culture*

A supportive system that promotes nurse and nursing faculty well-being was described as having positive relationships that align the person, family, community, and role as a nurse. The support system should be both at work and at home. Well-being is further provided through a work culture that is blame-free, which allows nurses and nursing faculty to work and live without fear. Institutions can support well-being by implementing policies to ensure healthy nurses, providing resources to nurses and nursing faculty, opening relaxation spaces at work, and providing opportunities to thrive and find harmony. Additional strategies include having a tolerable workload, reducing administrative burden, having a voice and being heard in the workplace, and networking. These strategies allow nurses and nursing faculty to navigate the ups and downs of practice. Systems and institutions also can incorporate Swarbrick's (2023) eight dimensions of wellness (i.e., physical, spiritual, emotional, social, environmental, intellectual, financial, occupational).

### *Personal Growth and Self-Awareness*

Personal growth and self-awareness were represented as being able to "show up" authentically, being one's true self in all settings and all interactions. Internal attributes for this category of well-being were depicted as being happy, having a sense of positivity, being content with personal life, celebrating oneself, having inner peace, and letting go. Attributes visible to others included being open to change, striving to be better and thrive, having a strong sense of self, living with a sense of abundance versus scarcity, and demonstrating resilience in times of stress and change.

### Positive Outcomes and Broader Impact

Discussants provided examples of how well-being could be measured. For example, a nursing program could measure student success and faculty retention as positive indicators of well-being. A clinical agency could monitor positive patient outcomes as a measure of nurse well-being. More generally, well-being could be identified as nurses and nursing faculty serving as role models, being impactful at work, and making contributions to patients, families, colleagues, and society. In addition, national nursing associations could access findings from the World Happiness Report as a proxy for nurse well-being.

## Barriers to Nurse and Nursing Faculty Well-Being

There are nine themes that describe the barriers to nurse and nursing faculty well-being. The themes are Leadership and Organizational Support, Workload and Staffing, Mental Health and Emotional Well-Being, Communication and Relationships, Resources and Infrastructure, Recognition and Value, Training and Education, Policy and Systemic Issues, and Personal and Social Factors.

### Leadership and Organizational Support

Leadership directly impacts well-being. For example, a lack of leadership or organizational support from all levels where profit and other outcomes are prioritized over best practice and the people completing the work (e.g., nurses, nursing faculty) can lead to negative well-being. In some instances, efforts may be implemented, but there is no organizational visibility and intention with the activities. There also may be new leaders to the organization, poor role modeling (e.g., leaders not role modeling well-being behaviors), lack of awareness and understanding, or lack of accountability.

### Workload and Staffing

The ongoing nursing and nursing faculty shortage across the globe contributes to high workload demands. For nurses, this also could mean a lack of choice in shifts. For nursing faculty, this contributes to feeling obligated to respond to students around the clock (e.g., all hours of the day/night, every day of the week). These work expectations then override time for work-life balance activities. Additional stressors contributing to negative nursing faculty well-being are administrative burdens and expectations to achieve promotion and tenure. Additional negative factors include the increasing complexity of demands and effort needed to do simple tasks, having more responsibility with less authority, and a shortage of nurses and/or faculty members that may lack the necessary skill set.

### Mental Health and Emotional Well-Being

Nurses and nursing faculty have minimal time to decompress or seek help. This results in an increase in focusing on the negative aspects of workload. This negative messaging can lead to substance use disorder, lack of self-care, stigma of not working hard enough, and playing the "victim." Some nurses do not know how to get help when needed, are afraid to speak out about issues or offer solutions, or do not seek professional help due to fear of regulatory boards. These negative aspects of mental health and emotional well-being can lead a group to think that burnout is normal, the spreading of anxiety within a work group, and loss of empathy towards those who are struggling.

### *Communication and Relationships*

The social hierarchy in health care can negatively impact well-being. It can contribute to a lack of peer support, difficulty in making work friends, and poor relationships. As the work environment deteriorates, behaviors such as incivility, cyberbullying, inability to set appropriate boundaries, escalation of interpersonal violence, and bias against people who are thriving can become normalized. This environment then becomes the axiom of nurses "eating their young."

### *Resources and Infrastructure*

Although resources and infrastructure could support a healthy work environment, the lack of funding for well-being initiatives is a challenge. Ongoing budget cuts have created an environment with limited internal and external resources, leading to unreasonable expectations given available resources. Other factors related to resources and infrastructure include a lack of break and rest areas, the rapid evolution of technology, and the costs of solving the challenges faced by nurses and nursing faculty. In addition, some discussants reported an ongoing shortage of personal protective equipment in their country.

### *Recognition and Value*

Nurses and nursing faculty are not valued as they should be. There is decreased recognition of their work, low wages, and a lack of well-being initiatives for nurses and nursing faculty. In addition, there is a lack of non-nurses to advocate for nurses, and nursing remains medically dominated.

### *Training and Education*

Nursing curricula remain overloaded, which impacts the workload of nursing faculty. Unfortunately, nurse well-being is not a common topic in nursing curricula. Thus, there is no preparation for managing stressful clinical situations (e.g., neonatal death). Also, there is a lack of knowledge about how to obtain help when needed, and no incentives for lifelong learning.

### *Policy and Systemic Issues*

There is no organizational visibility or intention for nurse and nursing faculty well-being. This lack of organizational priority is visible in systems that do not support nurses and nursing faculty questioning or challenging the status quo, that do not follow their purpose and mission (e.g., misaligned organization), and that exclude topics of bias from their policies. Systemic issues further occur through conflict-avoidant and/or toxic leadership and viewing well-being as something extra rather than fundamental. At a national level, political interference coupled with a devaluing of nursing and higher education also may contribute. These challenges lead nurses and nursing faculty to blame the system.

### *Personal and Social Factors*

On a personal level, nurses and nursing faculty perceive a lack of time and opportunity for self-development, rely heavily on their employment and fear a loss of their job, feel unable to say "no," and have a self-responsibility mindset. Socially, nurses and nursing faculty may have poor relationships, social isolation, changing family structure, and high personal social demands. These challenges, which are exacerbated by personal ego, martyrdom fixed complex, not recognizing that there is a problem, and fear of damage to reputation, lead nurses and nursing faculty to deprioritize themselves, thus resulting in poor well-being.

## Proposed Solutions for a Healthy Work Environment

There are nine themes that recommend proposed solutions to create sustainable, healthy work environments where students, nurses, and nursing faculty can thrive. The themes are Education and Curriculum, Well-Being and Mental Health, Leadership and Governance, Support Systems and Resources, Workplace Environment, Equity and Inclusion, Communication and Collaboration, Recognition and Motivation, and Technology and Innovation.

### *Education and Curriculum*

Strategies for supporting well-being are needed for nurses and nursing faculty. Nursing faculty can prepare students for realistic work to reduce future mismatched expectations as a nurse, teach students how to redesign systems, and embed general well-being topics into curricula. Systems can invest in role orientation of new hires (e.g., nurses, nursing faculty) to promote retention, require individual self-care time, and promote a human-centered organizational design. In general, nurses and nursing faculty can acknowledge caring science and participate in training opportunities on conflict de-escalation, mindfulness, and finance and economics to increase pay and obtain fees for services.

### *Well-Being and Mental Health*

Nurses and nursing faculty need to change their mindset and permit themselves to dream. They need to be aware of their fight-or-flight response when stressed and respond in a healthy manner, including determining what helps them achieve a healthy balance. Strategies to further promote their well-being and mental health include using dedicated well-being spaces and participating in dialectical behavior therapy or supportive counseling.

## *Leadership and Governance*

Leadership can promote nurse and faculty well-being by noting positive observed behaviors as well as areas for growth in annual performance reviews/evaluations, enforcing policies consistently, ensuring a safe work environment, adhering to the organizational mission and vision, making well-being a strategic priority/pillar, increasing salaries, and being transparent in faculty salaries. Sustained well-being can be promoted by adopting shared governance models, implementing an institutional policy to promote health, assessing leadership competencies, being accountable, providing executive leadership coaching, and focusing on succession planning. In addition, nurses and nursing faculty should study positive deviants locally and globally for implementation.

## *Support Systems and Resources*

Well-being strategies vary from individual to system levels. Individually, nurses and nursing faculty can obtain support from family, social networks, work colleagues, and others. Interpersonally, nurses and nursing faculty can provide social and psychological support to their colleagues and help them identify their own well-being strategies. At the organization level, organizations can adopt well-being frameworks such as the U.S. Surgeon General's (2022) Five Essentials for Workplace Mental Health & Well-Being to promote nurse and nursing faculty well-being. They also can encourage mentor-mentee relationships; launch formal mentorship programs; provide resources and workshops, mindfulness training, and chair yoga; offer substance use education and education on how to get help; ensure adequate staffing; appoint a wellness coach; provide funding for basic needs; and integrate and focus on sustainable approaches and practices. Nationally, accreditors can incorporate well-being initiatives into their expectations.

## *Workplace Environment*

Well-being in the workplace could be positively impacted by dedicating spaces for well-being, prioritizing health in the workplace (e.g., exercise, nutrition), discussing positives and solutions in addition to problems, and allowing people to hug if they are comfortable with it. Nurses and nursing faculty can stop assuming that incivility, workplace violence, and burnout are normal; create charters for civility expectations; and co-create rules for safety. Organizations also can implement ethics committees as a place to raise concerns, offer violence prevention training, invest in workforce development, conduct pulse and climate surveys, and implement best practices. For nursing programs, academic administrators can work with school/college/university leaders to provide a dedicated dormitory for nursing students. In clinical practice, organizational leaders can allow nurses to vary their work assignments and offer a break from their regular work.

## *Equity and Inclusion*

All individuals should be included equitably in well-being efforts. This necessitates a fair and equitable distribution of workload. To accomplish this, workload should be reassessed on a regular basis, and structures should be more inclusive. Inclusion should go beyond racial diversity to include gender sensitivity and other forms of diversity, such as acceptance and openness to other points of view. There also should be a system in place that allows for independence, autonomy, and academic freedom.

### Communication and Collaboration

Student-faculty teams can collaborate to focus on mutual well-being. Teams with nurses can identify meaningful solutions. Nurses and nursing faculty should prioritize teamwork, interprofessional collaboration, come together to lobby for more resources, create teams for community belonging, continue to bring problems forward, and promote healthy partnerships and good relationships. Well-being also can be promoted by listening to each other; using clear, transparent communication; calling out "gaslighting;" and using feedback loops.

### Recognition and Motivation

Recognition of nurses and nursing faculty is necessary to enhance motivation and ultimately well-being. Initially, nurses and nursing faculty can take pride in themselves and their work, focus on the competencies they have achieved rather than those they have not, implement gratitude circles, and change the narrative from negative to positive. Nursing and teaching need to be valued at all levels (e.g., by administrators, by politicians) and recognized for their work. This value and recognition can be demonstrated by increasing nursing faculty salaries; recognizing all positives, even small ones; creating opportunities to have fun; and nominating nurses and nursing faculty for Daisy Awards and other recognition programs.

### Technology and Innovation

A benefit of technology, innovation, and the use of AI is that it can reduce administrative burden and free up time for meaningful human connections. Further development of apps and short videos can be used to promote happiness and healthy lifestyles.

## CONCLUSION

Nurse and nursing faculty well-being is critical for the sustainability of the workforce. Well-being can be demonstrated by a sense of professional fulfillment and meaning and a positive work-life balance. Discussants reported multiple barriers that negatively impact nurse and nursing faculty well-being including a lack of effective leadership and organizational support, shortstaffing, excessive workload, toxic work relationships, and a lack of recognition for the work that nurses and nursing faculty do. Discussants recommended a variety of strategies to overcome these challenges such as training and education, positive relationships, and recognition of the value and work of nursing as a discipline.

## *References*

Bembridge, E., Crowfoot, G., Wilson, R., & Reis, J. (2025). Digital reflective practice among new graduate nurses—A scoping review. *Nurse Education Today*, *150*, 106688. https://doi.org/10.1016/j.nedt.2025.106688

Black, I. E., Perry, L., & Lee, H. (2025). Holistic wellness support systems for nursing faculty: A scoping review of the literature. *Nursing Education Perspectives*, *46*(1), 25–29. https://doi.org/10.1097/01.NEP.0000000000001277

Brodie, L., (2026). iCare Compassionately: A model for integrating compassionate care into nursing education. *Nurse Educator, 51*(1), e52–e57. http://doi.org/10.1097/NNE.0000000000002036

Grubaugh, M., Africa, L., & Neisinger, K. (2023). Managing the current workforce: Status of new graduate nurse well-being and clinical development 2018-2021. *Nursing Administration Quarterly*, *47*(3), 257–268. https://doi.org/10.1097/NAQ.0000000000000585

National League for Nursing Civil and Healthy Academic Work Environment Strategic Action Group. (2018, September). *NLN vision statement: Creating community to build a civil and healthy academic work environment*. National League for Nursing. https://www.nln.org/docs/default-source/uploaded-files/professional-development-programs/vision-statement-a-vision-for-creating-community-to-build-a-civil-and-healthy.pdf?sfvrsn=2ca7ab0d_0&pdf=VisionSeries-CreatingCommunity

Snow, F., Brown, L. M., & Scheller, S. (2024). The power of nursing: Person-centered self-care education for student nurses. *Holistic Nursing Practice*, *38*(5), 252–258. https://doi.org/10.1097/HNP.0000000000000656

Swarbrick, M. (2023). *The evolution of the wellness model*. Collaborative Support Programs of New Jersey. https://cspnj.org/wp-content/uploads/2024/02/Wellness-Model-Evolution-2023-1.pdf

U.S. Surgeon General. (2022). *The U.S. Surgeon General's framework for workplace mental health & well-being.* U.S. Department of Health and Human Services. https://www.hhs.gov/sites/default/files/workplace-mental-health-well-being.pdf

Zangaro, G. A., Leaver, C., & Rosseter, R. (2025). A measure of wellness among nursing faculty. *Journal of Professional Nursing, 57*, 68–74. https://doi.org/10.1016/j.profnurs.2025.01.008

PART 6

# Addressing the Global Nursing Faculty Shortage

12

# Overview of the Global Nursing Faculty Shortage

**Nuhad Yazbik Dumit, Patricia A. Sharpnack,
Erna Snelgrove-Clarke, and Ann Bonner**

## INTRODUCTION

Nurse educators are essential to building the future nursing workforce. Yet the global nursing faculty shortage is an international concern as it overlaps with the growing demand for qualified nurses. According to AACN, there are approximately 2,000 full-time faculty vacancies across the United States alone, with many institutions needing to create additional faculty positions to accommodate student demand (Byrne et al., 2023). Aging faculty, impending retirements, global migration, and inability to fill vacant positions due to workload, compensation, and devaluation of the educator's role are major factors contributing to the shortage. The example that follows represents the current reality for many novice nurse educators. We share this story with the goal of highlighting these experiences and bring to life the concerns for the international nurse educator shortage.

> *Maria graduated with a Bachelor of Nursing degree from her local university. Not only was she excited to provide nursing care to the many patients in her city, she also was dreaming of the day she too would be able to educate others to be nurses. During her education, Maria often heard rumblings of the nurse educator shortage, the many demands of the role, the poor pay, and lack of adequate orientation. She wondered about the accuracy of these stories and did not want to believe these were representative of the world of nurse educators. When Maria finally got her dream position to be a faculty member at her local university, she quickly discovered these "stories" to be true.*

In this chapter, we address the nursing faculty shortage, discuss advancing diversity of nursing faculty, and provide models and strategies to increase the nursing faculty workforce. We conclude with several practices that promote excellence and sustainability of nursing faculty. Like Maria, we strive to support the continued essence of nursing through clinical practice, education, research, and leadership.

## CHALLENGES DRIVING THE NURSING FACULTY SHORTAGE

The global shortage of qualified nursing faculty is a complex and multifaceted issue that significantly threatens the quality and sustainability of nursing education programs. Central to this challenge are persistent concerns regarding the pedagogical preparedness of nurse educators, limited access to professional development, and inadequate institutional support (Spector et al., 2020). These factors contribute to declining program quality, reduced student learning outcomes, and a diminished capacity to educate the next generation of nurses.

Knowledge of basic education pedagogy serves as an indicator of quality education outcomes, recruitment, and retention of nursing faculty (National Advisory Council on Nursing Education and Practice, 2021). The NCSBN studied nursing education program performance finding a statistically significant difference between those programs that maintained full nursing board approval and those programs that lost approval (Spector et al., 2020). A contributing factor to this lower quality in nursing programs was that there were more faculty who had not undertaken formal training in nursing education pedagogies (Spector et al., 2020). Furthermore, according to Antig et al. (2024), the shortage of faculty—both in numbers and depth of experience—negatively impacts the learning of students.

Researchers that explored faculty preparedness for their role show challenges in recruitment and retention of nurse educators that are influenced by several factors including unpreparedness for the faculty role; lack of professional development opportunities, competitive salaries, and low compensation; working environments that include unrealistic workload and poor collegial relationships; and lack of appreciation and recognition of faculty efforts and successes (Anderson et al., 2024; Bakewell-Sachs et al., 2022; Han et al., 2022; Vagharseyyedin & Sabeghi, 2025). In addition, findings of the AACN 2021 survey of nursing schools concluded that faculty shortages were caused by a lack of faculty with the right specialty mix and a limited pool of doctorally prepared faculty. Moreover, the survey showed major reasons for the faculty shortage include lack of funding to hire more full-time faculty and that there is significant competition from better paying clinical practice positions (AACN, 2021). On the other hand, studies show that the leading motivators for faculty retention are the passion to work with students, the belief in their ability to shape the nursing profession, a positive work environment that fosters collegial relationships and flexibility, and effective mentorship (Clochesy et al., 2019).

Despite these persistent challenges in recruitment and retention, research also highlights promising motivators and initiatives aimed at strengthening faculty preparedness. Strategies to prepare nursing faculty include integrating the scholarship of teaching in doctoral education and other graduate curricula (Han et al., 2022)—such as the New Jersey Nursing Initiative Faculty Preparation Program for doctoral students, the University of Louisiana's Program of Nursing Teacher-Scholar Project, and the Institute for Nursing Faculty Recruitment, Retention and Mentoring (INFORM). Initiatives are needed that "... supports efforts to eliminate the perspective divide between research and clinical faculty and build a common approach to scholarship and citizenship" (Clochesy et al., 2019, p. 63).

Antig et al. (2024) found that students reported challenges with learning platforms, delivery of instruction, and clinical experiences, and struggled to develop critical thinking and reasoning skills due to the shortage of qualified educators. To be effective, an educator must understand learning theories, curriculum development, assessment, and evaluation. Mastering this complexity takes time and is comparable to the transition from student to professional nurse (Speck et al., 2025). A commitment to lifelong learning is essential for nursing faculty to remain effective educators and leaders in the specialty of nursing education (Clochesy et al., 2019; Halstead & Frank, 2017; Han et al., 2022; Ramirez et al., 2022; Vagharseyyedin & Sabeghi, 2025).

The nursing faculty shortage also has affected the availability of places in nursing programs, forcing qualified applicants (students) to be turned away. Reduced admission capacity to nursing programs directly impacts the pipeline of new nurses entering the workforce. AACN (2024) reported that nursing programs turned away more than 65,000 qualified applicants from baccalaureate and graduate nursing programs in 2023 due to an insufficient number of faculty, clinical sites, classroom space, clinical preceptors, and budget constraints: citing the nursing faculty shortage as the top reason for not accepting all qualified applicants. The shortage of nursing faculty to educate future generations of nurses is likely to expand without coordinated initiatives to mitigate this gap. There remains a critical need and moral imperative for the profession and key interested parties across the world to address the nursing faculty shortage to reduce the effect it will have on the quality and availability of future health care. Targeted and bold initiatives are essential to reverse this trend.

## ADVANCING DIVERSITY IN NURSE EDUCATOR FACULTY

Globally, diversity among nursing faculty is essential because it enhances educational outcomes, fosters innovation, and reflects the pluralistic societies that institutions serve. A diverse nursing faculty contributes to improved student retention and success, particularly among underrepresented groups, by offering relatable role models and inclusive pedagogical approaches (Education Trust, 2022). Nursing programs with diverse nursing faculty are likely to be better equipped to address complex global challenges. Addressing the systemic barriers of recruiting nursing faculty is critical for institutions aiming to cultivate equitable and dynamic academic environments.

Diversity in faculty refers to the representation and inclusion of individuals from varied backgrounds, such as race, ethnicity, gender, age, disability, sexual orientation, socioeconomic status, and cultural heritage (Griffith University, 2025). Diversity encompasses both visible and invisible differences that shape perspectives and experiences within academic environments. The diversity of faculty also should reflect the broader society in which the academic environment is situated, as it will enrich institutional culture, academic excellence, and student experiences (Gasman et al., 2015).

In nursing, faculty diversity remains limited across multiple countries. AACN (2023) reported that in the United States, only 19.2 percent of full-time nursing faculty identify as minorities and just 7.4 percent as male. A review by Lartey et al. (2025) highlights that diverse faculty are vital for culturally competent education and student engagement, but that substantial barriers remain. Despite attempting to grow racial diversity in the nursing workforce, educator roles remain disproportionately White (Sandhu & Liao, 2024).

Beyond the United States, studies from Australia, Canada, and the United Kingdom reveal parallel trends. In Australia, the lack of culturally and linguistically diverse (CALD) faculty limits student cultural competence and feelings of isolation among First Nations (Indigenous) and migrant students (Candelaria et al., 2025). In Canada, students from CALD backgrounds report diminished sense of belonging and engagement when faculty are not representative of the multi-cultural society (dela Cruz et al., 2025; Lane et al., 2024). United

Kingdom–based research indicates that curricula often reflect a dominance of whiteness, which affects student identity formation and inclusive care delivery (Moorley & West, 2022).

Lack of diversity has tangible effects on students. Underrepresented nursing students may experience racism, discrimination, and a reduced sense of belonging—compromising their academic confidence and retention. The absence of relatable role models such as being taught by faculty from diverse backgrounds hinders professional identity development (Ganek et al., 2023). In Canada and Australia, for instance, students from diverse backgrounds often perceive lower levels of curricular inclusion and support, which can negatively influence their preparedness for clinical practice (dela Cruz et al., 2025; Lartey et al., 2025). Globally, the consequences are profound: students may be less equipped to serve diverse populations, and institutions risk reinforcing inequities in health care education.

Across the United States, Canada, and Australia, First Nations nursing academics are critically underrepresented, with serious implications for First Nations students. In Australia, Bonner et al. (2025) found that many universities lack First Nations faculty entirely, while those employed are often situated in junior roles despite advanced qualifications. The Canadian Association of Schools of Nursing (2023) survey highlights systemic barriers such as racism and inadequate mentorship that limit First Nations faculty participation and leadership. In the United States, programs such as the Native Nations Nursing Summit, along with initiatives elsewhere, are designed to support American Indian/Alaska Native scholars, yet their presence in academia remains marginal (University of Wisconsin–Madison, 2025). The exclusion of First Nations nurses may impede the creation of culturally safe learning environments and contribute to student disengagement, isolation, and inequities in academic support. Without First Nations role models and mentors, First Nations nursing students also may lack affirmation of their identities and aspirations within health care education, undermining both their academic success and broader health equity efforts.

To address these challenges, nursing faculty leaders must adopt inclusive and strategic reforms (Rhoten et al., 2024). As an initial strategic step, evaluating the faculty diversity profile to benchmark against the local population profile could inform a strategic diversity plan for the faculty to reach population parity. Faculty leaders must consistently communicate and role model the importance of equity, diversity, and inclusivity to support underrepresented minority faculty. Furthermore, strategic faculty diversity plan initiatives could include revising recruitment practices to attract diverse candidates, establishing mentorship programs, and engaging with minority-serving institutions and community organizations (ANA, 2023; Lartey et al., 2025). Hiring-selection panels to support the inclusion of diverse representation is needed, and those appointed to panels ought to have undertaken unconscious bias as well as cultural safety training. Faculty leaders also should embed diversity and equity within institutional structures through equity, diversity, and inclusivity committees; leadership training in cultural humility; and curricula reforms. All faculty should undertake cultural competence and anti-racism training as essential components of faculty development (Bonner et al., 2025). Lastly, mentorship and development of underrepresented faculty are required to provide professional support and appropriate workload profiles to increase faculty retention and assist with career advancement through promotion (Lartey et al., 2025). These interventions collectively enhance institutional workplace culture and attract, retain, and graduate nursing students from diverse backgrounds to enter the profession and deliver equitable and culturally safe care.

## MODELS AND STRATEGIES TO INCREASE AND DEVELOP THE NURSING FACULTY WORKFORCE

To address the global shortage of nursing faculty and increase this workforce, innovative strategies are urgently needed across both the education and health care sectors. Many nurses currently working in clinical positions are often interested in transitioning to academia, yet may hesitate to make a full-time shift. These nurses also may be unaware of the opportunities available. Expanding the nursing faculty workforce requires a concerted effort to make academic roles more accessible, flexible, and sustainable—while enhancing workforce diversity. Innovative strategies are needed to support recruitment and retention of qualified faculty (Heidari et al., 2024).

### Pathways for Nurses to Transition Into Academia

The transition from clinical practice to being a full-time nursing faculty member is often challenging for nurses as they must adapt to a very different work environment (Barrow & Xu, 2021). It involves a shift from being an expert clinician to that of novice faculty member. There is also a shift from patient care to understanding and applying teaching pedagogy, curriculum implementation, student rather than patient interaction, undertaking research, expectations to publish, and other faculty activities (Speck et al., 2025). Barken and Robstad (2024) in a study of nursing faculty in Norway described the transition as shifting from being clinically confident to being academically uncertain. An extended orientation and academic-career development pathway informed by the NLN's nurse educator core competencies could assist with the transition into the academic role (Christensen & Simmons, 2026).

One of the major barriers to becoming a faculty member is having the requisite qualifications. In many countries, faculty are expected to hold a qualification higher than the program in which they will be teaching. For instance, holding a master's or doctoral qualification to teach a bachelor's degree (East et al., 2024). In master's and doctoral programs, there needs to be opportunities to learn about pedagogy and curriculum and to acquire learning and teaching competencies. Other short-term programs such as microcredentials could accelerate the transition for advanced practice nurses who already hold master's or doctoral qualifications to enable them to move into faculty roles.

### Flexible and Part-Time Faculty Positions

As the clinical nursing workforce evolves—with more nurses seeking varied and adaptable work schedules—educational institutions also must offer greater flexibility in faculty positions (Moyer, 2022). Where institutional policies allow, supporting part-time (fractional) appointments rather than only full-time positions can help accommodate faculty with family or personal commitments that prohibit a full-time faculty position. Another effective strategy is implementing flexible work arrangements that combine on-campus and remote work activities. Hybrid models applied across teaching, research, and other organizational commitments not only support work-life balance but also enhance employee engagement with the organization, boost productivity, and improve staff retention (Moyer, 2022).

## Faculty Mentorship

Mentoring new nursing faculty is extremely important and should be a high priority for all nursing programs as a strategy to retain new nursing faculty members (Ephraim, 2021; Fernández-Lorente et al., 2025; Vagharseyyedin & Sabeghi, 2025) and to improve the likelihood of successful transition into academia for clinical nurses (Calaguas, 2023). It is common for many nursing programs to have formal (allocated mentors) or informal (mentees seek out mentors) mentorship strategies. In either situation, the quality of the relationship between the mentee and mentor could be an important factor in retaining new nursing faculty (Busby et al., 2022; Ephraim, 2021; Wyllie et al., 2019). One mentorship strategy could be to establish a structured bespoke mentorship program whereby the mentee identifies, with the assistance of a faculty mentor, the areas in which specific guidance is needed. Bespoke mentorship could involve navigating academic career paths, balancing clinical and academic responsibilities, and developing research and leadership skills. This bespoke approach is likely to need more than one faculty mentor. Emotional support, guidance, collaboration, and peer interactions can positively impact new faculty members' job satisfaction, productivity, and future career progression (Solberg et al., 2024).

In a recent review of mentoring practices for skills needed to teach nursing, Fernandez-Lorente et al. (2025) reported many benefits and positive impacts for mentorship and the development of new faculty. Through mentoring, the supportive transition into faculty roles revealed improved faculty retention, as well as personal and professional development, as potential outcomes of success. For example, focusing on teaching and learning strategies requires a supportive environment. Despite clinical expertise, many new educators have minimal educational pedagogy and classroom teaching experience. Attention needs to be given to the onboarding of these new educators (Wolsey & Jacobsen, 2024), as well as continued support and development for learning and incorporating a plethora of teaching and learning strategies (Satoh et al., 2024). Time for both professional development and mentoring is a necessary ingredient for success.

## Foster a Supportive and Inclusive Workplace Climate

Nursing education leaders and administrators have a crucial role in creating and fostering a supportive and inclusive climate, such as clearly communicating expectations, policies, and decision-making processes. These could be considered on an individual basis to best meet faculty needs, including initiatives to identify and address workplace biases and promote cultural sensitivity, and opportunities for nursing faculty to connect with colleagues within and outside their department (El-Banna et al., 2025; Everett, 2020). Other approaches could include establishing formal and informal mentorship programs to guide novice faculty and building a strong support network (Clochesy et al., 2019; Fernandez-Lorente et al., 2025; Koenig, 2019).

## Clinical Faculty Partnerships and Shared Appointments

Another strategy is to create clinical faculty positions situated across both educational institutions and health care services. This strategy is attractive to many nurses, because they can maintain their clinical practice through providing direct patient care while also undertaking teaching. These positions tend to be created as a partnership between education and health organizations and enable experienced clinical nurses to teach part-time or as adjuncts, without leaving their clinical careers entirely (Polancich et al., 2021). Nurses employed in these partnership positions often focus their teaching in the nursing laboratories, where their recent clinical practice experiences enrich the simulated learning environment. Nursing students often view expert clinicians as role models because of their currency of clinical practice (Speck et al., 2025).

Shared (joint) appointments are an alternative model whereby nurses hold faculty positions at academic institutions while also working at hospitals or other health care facilities. These positions are typically created for research purposes and research-capacity building of clinical nurses and are often embedded in academic-clinical partnerships (Albert et al., 2022; Allen et al., 2023). These shared positions may be divided equally in time and/or responsibilities (50 percent in each organization) or some other variation (Lauck et al., 2022). In some situations, both organizations contribute funding for the position. While often at the professor level (Pattison et al., 2022), increasingly shared (joint) positions can be across the academic career trajectory—commencing with early-career academics to senior levels (Johnson et al., 2023). Joint appointments ensure that nursing faculty stay connected to real-world health care and can undertake novel research, including knowledge translation into practice.

## CONTRIBUTING TO EXCELLENCE AND SUSTAINABILITY OF NURSING FACULTY

In our experience as nurse leaders, several practices contribute to excellence and sustainability in nursing faculty. When working predominantly with novice nursing faculty, person-centered leadership style enables both the leader and the faculty to be value-focused. There is a need to provide support that aligns with the faculty's needs while striving to create a sense of belonging. This relational approach to leadership supports effective workplace cultures and flourishing (Cardiff et al., 2018). Mutual respect and understanding, in a bidirectional approach, strengthen work relationships.

Nursing faculty effectiveness is evidenced when leadership is relational. Excellence and sustainability in faculty development are evident when leaders work with the principles of collaboration, inclusion, and participation (Hardy et al., 2021; Martin, 2023). Meeting regularly with faculty, including faculty in decision-making, and challenging one another with strong support empower faculty. These approaches support a shared vision and a goal of faculty wellness and success. Faculty see a leader as being authentic when they are open, patient, and optimistic. Faculty perceive that they are heard when a leader practices authentic listening. Person-centered participatory action leadership research conducted by Cardiff et al. (2018) concluded that a person-centered approach to leadership fosters healthful relationships and growth. Relational leadership can result in higher performance, excellence, and sustainability in nursing faculty. Working with faculty and for faculty supports their academic endeavors.

Working within existing structures can be challenging, and it is often necessary to build trusting relationships. A leader's role modeling of their values provides an opportunity for new and experienced nursing faculty to observe and even acknowledge a leader's behaviors. Encouraging and welcoming feedback from nursing faculty creates a culture of inclusion and a willingness to work together for personal and professional growth.

## INTERNATIONAL COUNCIL OF NURSES

ICN, in collaboration with NLN, has identified the global nursing faculty shortage as a critical issue requiring urgent attention. Recognizing that the nursing faculty workforce impacts the global preparation of the future nursing workforce, a subcommittee of the ICN Education Experts Advisory Committee developed a policy brief to address this challenge. Although the ICN has not yet released the policy brief, the authors of this chapter were members of the subcommittee. The policy brief was informed by a comprehensive literature review and explored key themes, including the roles of nurse educators, causes of the faculty shortage, and potential solutions. It emphasizes the importance of policy action at both national and international levels to strengthen nurse educator competencies and ensure a sustainable nursing faculty workforce. The brief also includes a set of evidence-based recommendations focused on improving faculty recruitment, strengthening faculty retention, enhancing faculty development, and aligning nurse educator capabilities with evolving health system needs.

## CONCLUSION

Addressing the global nursing faculty shortage demands a multifaceted and forward-thinking approach involving individuals, faculty, and leaders, as well as the broader profession. Without sufficient nursing faculty, the global nursing workforce shortage will continue to expand. This chapter has explored that the nursing faculty workforce is enriched by its diversity, which must be actively cultivated and supported through inclusive policies and practices. Nursing programs are uniquely positioned to lead this transformation by adopting innovative, alternative models that not only expand pathways for nurses to transition into academia but also reimagine faculty roles through flexible, part-time, and shared appointments with hospitals and other health services.

Mentorship programs, inclusive workplace cultures, and strategic clinical-academic partnerships are essential components in building a sustainable and resilient nursing faculty workforce. These strategies not only support nursing faculty retention and development but also contribute to the overall excellence of nursing education and to the preparation of the future nursing workforce. Importantly, fostering a climate of belonging and professional growth ensures that nursing faculty from varied backgrounds can thrive and contribute meaningfully to education, research, and clinical practice in the discipline.

To ensure these efforts are impactful and enduring, evaluation of implemented models, strategies, and policies is essential. Faculty leaders must commit to ongoing assessment, refinement, and dissemination of best practices to inform local, national, and international education providers. By doing so, a diverse, well-prepared, and adaptable nursing faculty workforce is in place to educate future generations of nurses—ultimately strengthening the profession and improving health outcomes worldwide.

## References

Albert, N. M., Chipps, E., Klein, C. J., Briskin, I., Falkenberg Olsen, A. C., Liu Hand, L., Harmon, M. M., Heitschmidt, M., & Talsma, A. (2022). A cross-sectional study of United States academic-clinical research collaborations: Characteristics, resources, benefits and outcomes. *Journal of Clinical Nursing*, *31*, 435–444. https://doi.org/10.1111/jocn.15597

Allen, D. H., Arthur, E. K., Blazey, M., Brassil, K., Cahill, J. E., Cooley, M. E., Fadol, A. P., Hammer, M. J., Hartranft, S., Murphy, B., Nolan, T. S., Sun, V., Whisenant, M., & Yoder, L. H. (2023). A scoping review on the nurse scientist role within healthcare systems. *Worldviews on Evidence-Based Nursing*, *20*, 47–55. https://doi.org/10.1111/wvn.12624

American Association of Colleges of Nursing. (2021). *2020-2021 Salaries of instructional and administrative nursing faculty in baccalaureate and graduate programs in nursing*. American Association of Colleges of Nursing.

American Association of Colleges of Nursing. (2023). *Enhancing diversity in the nursing workforce*. American Association of Colleges of Nursing. https://www.aacnnursing.org/news-data/fact-sheets/enhancing-diversity-in-the-nursing-workforce

American Association of Colleges of Nursing. (2024). *2023-2024 enrollment and graduations in baccalaureate and graduate programs in nursing.* American Association of Colleges of Nursing. https://www.aacnnursing.org/news-data/fact-sheets/nursing-faculty-shortage

American Nurses Association. (2023). *How nursing leaders can promote diversity in nursing*. American Nurses Association. https://www.nursingworld.org/content-hub/resources/workplace/promote-diversity-in-nursing/

Anderson M., Taylor N., Rowley T., Owens C., & Iacob E. (2024). Understanding factors influencing nursing faculty departure and intentions. *Nurse Educator*, *49*(4), 222–226. https://doi.org/10.1097/nne.0000000000001612

Antig, A., Arañez, S., Cañazares, C., & Palompon, D. (2024). Nursing faculty shortage impact on nursing students: A descriptive phenomenological study. *Nursing Research and Practice, 2024*, 1751942. https://doi.org/10.1155/2024/1751942

Bakewell-Sachs, S., Trautman, D., & Rosseter, R. (2022). *Addressing the nurse faculty shortage*. American Nurse. https://www.myamericannurse.com/addressing-the-nurse-faculty-shortage-2/

Barken, T. L., & Robstad, N. (2024). Academic nurses' transition across an academic career: A qualitative study. *Journal of Advanced Nursing*, *80*(4), 1630–1637. https://doi.org/10.1111/jan.15928

Barrow, M., & Xu, L. (2021). Making their way as academics: A qualitative study examining how nurse academics understand and (re) construct academic identity. *Nurse Education Today*, *100*, 104820. https://doi.org/10.1016/j.nedt.2021.104820

Bonner, A., Deravin, L., Dewar, J., Williamson, M., Gillespie, K., Atherfold, C., Nightingale, K., West, C., & Strickland, K. (2025). Aboriginal, Torres Strait Islander and Māori nursing and midwifery academic workforce across Australia and New Zealand. *Collegian*, *32*(3), 149–154. https://doi.org/10.1016/j.colegn.2025.03.004

Busby, K. R., Draucker, C. B., & Reising, D. L. (2022). Exploring mentoring and nurse faculty: An integrative review. *Journal of Professional Nursing*, *38*, 26–39. https://doi.org/10.1016/j.profnurs.2021.11.006

Byrne, C., Keyt, J., & Fang, D. (2023). *Special survey on vacant faculty positions for academic year 2022-2023.* American Association of Colleges of Nursing. https://www.aacnnursing.org/Portals/0/PDFs/Data/Vacancy23.pdf.

Calaguas, N. P. (2023). Mentoring novice nurse educators: Goals, principles, models, and key practices. *Journal of Professional Nursing*, *44*, 8–11. https://doi.org/10.1016/j.profnurs.2022.11.002

Candelaria, D., River, J., Gallagher, R., & McCormack, B. (2025). Harnessing the collective power of gender equity and diversity in nursing. *Journal of Advanced Nursing*, in press. https://doi.org/10.1111/jan.16835

Canadian Association of Schools of Nursing. (2023). *Indigenous nursing student and faculty survey report 2022–2023*. Canadian Association of Schools of Nursing. https://www.casn.ca/2024/12/indigenous-nursing-student-and-faculty-survey-report-2022-2023/

Cardiff, S., McCormack, B., & McCance, T. (2018). Person centred leadership: A relational approach to leadership derived through action research. *Journal of Clinical Nursing*, *15–16*, 3056–3069. https://doi.org/10.1111/jocn.14492

Christensen, L. S., & Simmons, L. E. (2026). *The scope of practice for academic nurse educators practicing in various academic nurse educator roles* (4th ed.). NLN Press.

Clochesy, J M., Visovsky, C., & Munro, CL. (2019). Preparing nurses for faculty roles: The Institute for Faculty Recruitment, Retention and Mentoring (INFORM), *Nurse Education Today*, *79*, 63–66. https://doi.org/10.1016/j.nedt.2019.05.018

dela Cruz, A., Odoko, K., Cummings, S., Ala, C., & Afzal, A. (2025). Equity, diversity and inclusion: Exploring Canadian nurses' perceptions. *Nursing Management, 32*(6). https://journals.rcni.com/doi/10.7748/nm.2025.e2159

East, L., Halcomb, E., Terry, D., Jackson, D., & Hutchinson, M. (2024). The Australian nursing and midwifery academic workforce: A cross-sectional study. *Nurse Education in Practice*, *81*, e104156. https://doi.org/10.1016/j.nepr.2024.104156

Education Trust. (2022). *Faculty diversity and student success go hand in hand*. Education Trust. https://edtrust.org/rti/faculty-diversity-and-student-success-go-hand-in-hand-so-why-are-university-faculties-so-white/

El-Banna, M. M., Alrimawi, I., Davis-Collins, K., & Rollins-Monroe, K. (2025). Recruiting and retaining diverse faculty and students: Strategies for success. *Teaching and Learning in Nursing*, *20*(3), 286–290. https://doi.org/10.1016/j.teln.2025.02.034

Ephraim, N. (2021). Mentoring in nursing education: An essential element in the retention of new nurse faculty. *Journal of Professional Nursing*, *37*(2), 306–319. https://doi.org/10.1016/j.profnurs.2020.12.001

Everett, M. C. (2020). Sharing the responsibility for nursing student retention. *Teaching and Learning in Nursing*, *15*(2), 121–122. https://doi.org/10.1016/j.teln.2019.12.009

Fernandez-Lorente, L., Rodriguez-Almagro, J., & Hernandez-Martinez, A. (2025). Enhancing support for new nursing faculty: An extensive scoping review of mentoring practices. *Nurse Education Today*, *147*, 106595. https://doi.org/10.1016/j.nedt.2025.106595

Ganek, E., Sazon, R. A. P., Gray, L., & Sherry, D. (2023). An introduction to faculty diversity, equity, and inclusion for excellence in nurse education: Literature review. *Asian/Pacific Island Nursing Journal*, *7*, e49231. http://dx.doi.org/10.2196/49231

Gasman, M., Abiola, U., & Travers, C. (2015). Diversity and senior leadership at elite institutions of higher education. *Journal of Diversity in Higher Education, 8*(1), 1–14. https://doi.org/10.1037/a0038872

Griffith University. (2025). *Staff equity, diversity and inclusion*. Griffith University. https://www.griffith.edu.au/equity

Halstead, J. A., & Frank, B. (2017). *Pathways to a Nursing Education Career*. Springer Publishing Company. https://connect.springerpub.com/content/book/978-0-8261-3999-3

Han, H. R., D'Aoust, R., Gross, D., Szanton, S., Nolan, M., Campbell, J., & Davidson, P. (2022). Preparing future nursing faculty: Integrating enhanced teaching and leadership development curricula into PhD education. *Journal of Advanced Nursing*, *78*(1), e3–e5. https://doi.org/10.1111/jan.14982

Hardy, S., Clarke, S., Frei, I., Morley, C., Odell, J., White, C., & Wilson, V. (2021). A global manifesto for practice development: Revisiting core principles. In K. Manley, V. Wilson, & C. Øye (Eds.), *International practice development in health and social care* (2nd ed., pp. 99–117). Wiley. https://doi.org/10.1002/9781119698463.ch8

Heidari, O., Adhia, A., Gondwe, K. W., Shin, M. B., Suárez-Baquero, D. F. M., & Ward, T. M. (2024). Experiences of recruitment and retention in academia: A collaborative autoethnography of early-career faculty members of color. *Nursing Outlook*, *72*(4), Article

102200. https://doi.org/10.1016/j.outlook.2024.102200

Johnson, M., Ferguson, C., Thornton, A., Israel, J., Cruickshank, M., Deboroah, D., Fernandez, R., Fry, M., Hickman, L. D., Hosie, A., Inglis, S. C., McErlean, G., McInnes, E., Perry, L., Sheppard-Law, S., Wynne, R., Parsons, M., & Middleton, S. (2023). Exploring the SPHERE nursing and midwifery clinician researcher career pathway: A qualitative study. *Collegian*, *30*(6), 795–804. https://doi.org/10.1016/j.colegn.2023.06.002

Koenig, A. M. (2019). Mentoring: Are we living up to our professional role as an educational leader? *Nurse Education Today*, *79*, 54–55. https://doi.org/10.1016/j.nedt.2019.04.007

Lane, J., Alizadeh, N., Daclan, A., & Vickery, A. (2024). Exploring the impact of equity, diversity, and inclusion initiatives within a Canadian nursing program: A pilot study. *Creative Nursing, 30*(3), 210–219. https://doi.org/10.1177/10784535241267944

Lartey, S. A., Cummings, G. G., Richter, S., & Montgomery, C. L. (2025). Equity, diversity and inclusion in nursing educational institutions: A scoping review. *Journal of Advanced Nursing,* in press. https://doi.org/10.1111/jan.17061

Lauck, S. B., Thorne, S. E., Saewyc, E. M., Heppell, L., Black, A. T., & Virani, S. A. (2022). Promoting cardiovascular nursing practice and research: A model for a university joint appointment. *Journal of Clinical Nursing*, *32*(3–4), 311–317. https://doi.org/10.1111/jocn.15588

Martin, D. (2023). *Engagement: The secret sauce to effective faculty professional development*. Faculty Focus. https://www.facultyfocus.com/articles/academic-leadership/engagement-the-secret-sauce-to-effective-faculty-professional-development/

Moorley, C., & West, R. (2022). Inclusivity in nurse education. *Evidence-Based Nursing*, *25*(3), 75–76. https://ebn.bmj.com/content/ebnurs/25/3/75.full.pdf

Moyer, S. M. (2022). Work-life balance of nursing faculty: A scoping review. *Nursing Education Perspectives*, *43*(4), 211–216. https://doi.org/10.1097/01.NEP.0000000000000952

National Advisory Council on Nursing Education and Practice. (2021). *Preparing nurse faculty and addressing the shortage of nurse faculty and clinical preceptors (report)*. Health Resources and Services Administration. https://www.hrsa.gov/sites/default/files/hrsa/advisory-committees/nursing/reports/nacnep-17report-2021.pdf

Pattison, N., Deaton, C., McCabe, C., Coates, V., Johnston, B., Nolan, F., & Briggs, M. (2022). Florence Nightingale's legacy for clinical academics: A framework analysis of a clinical professorial network and a model for clinical academia. *Journal of Clinical Nursing*, *31*(3–4), 353–361. https://doi.org/10.1111/jocn.15756

Polancich, S., Miltner, R., Poe, T., Harper, D., Moneyham, L., & Shirey, M. (2021). Innovations in evaluating nursing academic practice partnerships. *Journal of Nursing Administration, 51*(6), 347–353. https://doi.org/10.1097/NNA.0000000000001025

Ramirez, J., Ro, K., Lin, Y., Thomas, A., De Nysschen, M., Smart, A., & Robinson, G. (2022). Exploring alternative forms of scholarship for nurse educators' success. *Journal of Professional Nursing*, *43*, 68–73. https://doi.org/10.1016/j.profnurs.2022.09.001

Rhoten, B. A., Steed, J., Johnson, R., & Schorn, M. (2024). Evaluating and addressing the diversity, equity, inclusion, and belonging climate in a school of nursing. *Nurse Educator*, *49*(3), E153–E157. https://doi.org/10.1097/NNE.0000000000001529

Sandhu, R. D., & Liao, C. (2024). "In the end, we had to leave": Truth-telling to unsettle whiteness in nursing academia. *Nursing Outlook*, *72*(5), 102228. https://doi.org/10.1016/j.outlook.2024.102228

Satoh, M., Sato, N., Tamura, N., & Fujimura, A. (2024). Psychological safety in enhancing the competence of nurse educators among early career nursing faculty in Japan: A cross-sectional study. *International Journal of Nursing Studies Advances*, *7*, Article 100254. https://doi.org/10.1016/j.ijnsa.2024.100254

Solberg, M., Schlegel, E., Spurlock, E., Blair, L., & Nowak, A. (2024). Fostering Early Career Nursing Faculty Support in the Academy. *Nurse Educator, 49*(2), E97-E98. https://doi.org/10.1097/nne.0000000000001504

Speck, P. M., Milligan, G. W., Hammond, S. A., Hallman, M. G., & Steadman, L. A. (2025). An integrative literature review for the clinical expert transitioning to a nurse faculty role. *Journal of Professional Nursing*, *59*, 78–87. https://doi.org/10.1016/j.profnurs.2025.04.003

Spector, N., Silvesta, J., Alexander, M., Martin, B., Hooper, J. I., Squires, A., & Ojemeni, M. (2020). NCSBN regulatory guidelines and evidence-based quality indicators for nursing education programs. *Journal of Nursing Regulation, 11*(2), S1–S64. https://www.journalofnursingregulation.com/article/S2155-8256(20)30075-2/fulltext

University of Wisconsin–Madison. (2025). *Native Nations Nursing, Helpers, and Healers Summit*. University of Wisconsin–Madison. https://ce.icep.wisc.edu/content/2025-native-nations-nursing-helpers-and-healers-summit

Vagharseyyedin, S. A., & Sabeghi, H. (2025). Transition to the faculty role: A qualitative study into the experiences of nursing faculty. *Journal of Advances in Medical Education and Professionalism*, *13*(1), 59–66. https://pmc.ncbi.nlm.nih.gov/articles/PMC11788770/pdf/JAMP-13-59.pdf

Wolsey, C., & Jacobson, M. (2024). Novice nurse educator professional learning and teaching at a transnational nursing campus: A case study. *Nurse Education in Practice*, *79*, 104028. https://doi.org/10.1016/j.nepr.2024.104028

Wyllie, A., Levett-Jones, T., DiGiacomo, M., & Davidson, P. (2019). Exploring the experiences of early career academic nurses as they shape their career journey: A qualitative study. *Nurse Education Today*, *76*, 68–72. https://doi.org/10.1016/j.nedt.2019.01.021

# 13

# Barriers and Strategies for Addressing the Global Nursing Faculty Shortage

**Gordon Lee Gillespie and Sandra Davis**

## INTRODUCTION

In the United States, the overall vacancy rate of nursing faculty positions is 7.8 percent (Byrne et al., 2023). This nursing faculty shortage is just for the United States and does not take into account the prevalence of the problem globally. The leading reason for the nursing faculty shortage is a salary that is not competitive with those earned by nurses working in clinical practice settings (Byrne et al., 2023; Christianson et al., 2025). Other reasons for the inability to recruit nursing faculty include limited pool of doctorally prepared faculty, difficulty finding faculty willing to teach clinical courses, and heavy faculty workload (Byrne et al., 2023). Interventions are needed to address these problems so that nursing faculty can be recruited and retained. Initially, there needs to be multiple pathways for nurses to obtain the necessary competencies to become an effective nurse educator, such as formal degrees or certificate programs (Kerns & Wedgeworth, 2026). Expert nurses working in clinical practice settings can be recruited to serve in a dual appointment, with 10 percent of their time reallocated to teaching in the clinical setting where they currently practice as a nurse (Fitzpatrick & Forcina, 2026; Keenan et al., 2025). Expert nurses also can participate in formal nurse residency programs where they learn to become faculty members (Gazza et al., 2025). Once hired, new nursing faculty can partner with experienced faculty to co-teach courses (Calaguas, 2025), allowing experienced faculty to role model effective teaching while helping the new faculty member transition into the role. Transition to faculty programs has strong potential to increase nursing faculty satisfaction as well as faculty competency, retention, and academic achievements (Jones et al., 2026). International efforts such as the partnership between the ICN and NLN to form the ICN Expert Educators Advisory Committee can be leveraged to address the unique needs of faculty globally (Sharpnack, 2025).

## WORLD CAFÉ QUESTIONS

Following a panel on the global nursing faculty shortage, Utstein attendees responded to one of three questions at their various tables. After predetermined periods of time, they rotated to different tables allowing them to ultimately respond to all three questions. The three questions were:

1. What are the barriers and proposed solutions for recruiting and retaining nursing faculty in your country?
2. What strategies can be used to create nurse educator pathways in your country?
3. What strategies can be used to promote diversity of the faculty in your country?

This chapter describes the findings based on discussants' responses to the three questions on the global nursing faculty shortage. Details on the data collection procedures are described in Chapter 2.

## FINDINGS

### Barriers to Faculty Recruitment and Retention

There are five themes that depict barriers to recruiting and retaining faculty in discussants' countries. The themes are Compensation and Financial Disparities, Workload and Role Expectations, Career Pathway and Advancement Challenges, Cultural and Institutional Barriers, and Policy and Structural Issues.

### Compensation and Financial Disparities

The global nursing faculty shortage is plagued by a salary gap between clinical practice and academic appointments, which reflects nursing faculty being paid considerably less than both nurses working in hospital organizations and faculty members in other disciplines. In addition, nursing faculty members with an advanced practice credential earn less than their counterparts in clinical practice (e.g., nurse practitioners). The competition between clinical practice and academia for qualified nurses will continue to negatively impact recruitment and retention of qualified nursing faculty. Although the cost of higher education has escalated, there remains a lack of resources for nursing programs to put toward faculty pay. Nursing program leaders do not use a business mindset for faculty recruitment and retention, which is used in other disciplines for the recruitment and retention of faculty.

### Workload and Role Expectations

Nursing faculty tend to have multiple roles within a nursing program, including educator, mentor, and administrator. Although faculty are expected to be adept at all aspects of this multidimensional role, there is minimal flexibility to accomplish the workload. Discussants reported that there are rigid definitions of nursing faculty workload, which lead to faculty being burdened with an overload in their teaching and administrative assignments. Ultimately, there is a mismatch between individual faculty expectations and faculty's ability to meet the nursing program's mission.

### Career Pathway and Advancement Challenges

Although there is a global nursing faculty shortage, there is minimal preparation of future nurse educators with the skills and training needed to be successful. Also, there are either no incentives or nurses are dissatisfied with the incentives offered to them to become nursing faculty. Multiple programs require a minimum of a master of science to teach in a registered nurse program, which further limits the ability of undergraduate prepared nurses to teach the next generation of nurses. Once hired, it is difficult for nurses to transition into nursing faculty roles. There is inadequate preparation or support to advance between the faculty ranks or to attain tenure.

### Cultural and Institutional Barriers

There are multiple cultural and institutional barriers that prevent nurses from seeking nursing faculty positions. Discussants identified common problems as experiences of racism, lack of exposure to the role of teaching, negative image of nurse educators, teaching not seen as a distinct specialty practice, and poor workload. Similarly, they identified barriers to nursing faculty retention, including lack of nursing faculty status within the university setting, teaching-focused faculty not as respected or rewarded as research-focused faculty, pedagogical research not respected, and lack of available research funding.

### *Policy and Structural Issues*

Many nurses prefer working with patients versus students. Budget cuts in higher education make it difficult to recruit and sway these nurses to consider a position as a nursing faculty member. In addition, some countries have not ratified the International Labour Office's (2005) Nursing Personnel Convention (no. 149) describing the qualifications and roles of a registered nurse. This lack of adoption coupled with an emerging devaluation of higher education further limits nurses' desire to obtain a graduate degree to then become nursing faculty. Once hired, nursing faculty realize the need to practice clinically and conduct research, in addition to teaching, to obtain tenure. Without an academic practice role similar to academic medicine, nursing faculty find minimal support to be successful. In addition, some countries are experiencing political conflict, which contributes to a sense of insecurity and worsening emigration, further increasing that country's nursing faculty shortage.

## Solutions for Faculty Recruitment and Retention

There are five themes that depict solutions for recruiting and retaining faculty in discussants' countries. The themes are Financial Incentives and Support, Faculty Development and Mentorship, Flexibility and Innovative Work Models, Policy and Advocacy, and Recruitment and Retention Strategies.

### *Financial Incentives and Support*

The most frequent strategy recommended by discussants was to offer financial incentives for faculty recruitment and retention, particularly offering higher salaries to address the pay gap. Additional financial remunerations included start-up funding, research resources, compensation for certifications in teaching and learning, academic leave (e.g., sabbatical), and other benefits. Initiating faculty practice was mentioned as a strategy to increase faculty salary. Nursing faculty support also was discussed as grants, fellowships, and inducements to pursue a higher degree. Discussants recommended shifting the sponsorship of these costs to the end user (e.g., industry) and seeking funding from local businesses.

### *Faculty Development and Mentorship*

Faculty development and mentorship were key strategies to promote nursing faculty recruitment and retention. Faculty development includes offering teaching assistant positions, launching faculty residency programs, supporting certifications in teaching and learning, providing regular training on how to be an effective educator, and paying for professional conferences and leadership development programs focused on the role of a nurse educator (e.g., NLN Education Summit, NLN LEAD Program). Mentorship includes participating in formal mentorship programs, assisting faculty to be promoted, developing a professional development plan, and establishing faculty networks.

### Flexibility and Innovative Work Models

Nursing faculty need flexible schedules, time off, and a fair workload. Supportive efforts can include workload release to obtain terminal degrees; redistribution of workload percentage effort allocated to the tripartite mission of teaching, scholarship, and service; and implementation of new models to assign nursing faculty workload. In addition, work–life balance initiatives and opportunities for faculty practice roles can promote nursing faculty recruitment and retention.

### Policy and Advocacy

School administrators can conduct a strengths, weaknesses, opportunities, threats analysis to show local needs for improvement. General recommendations provided were improving the nursing program's budget, addressing the nursing faculty salary gap, adopting shared governance, establishing fair policies for promotion, and creating faculty practice partnerships. In addition, nursing faculty can advocate for policies/regulatory requirements to invest in the nurse faculty role and recommend common national policies for the nurse faculty role. The media can be leveraged to increase exposure of opportunities and benefits of being nursing faculty so that teaching is seen as more attractive.

### Recruitment and Retention Strategies

Recruitment efforts need to begin before students graduate from their nursing programs. Nursing faculty need to build a pipeline between academia and clinical practice and incorporate teaching and the nursing faculty role into doctoral programs. Nursing faculty also need to change the narrative to highlight the positive aspects of their work culture and role. In addition, funds need to be made available to support doctoral education for future nursing faculty. To retain nursing faculty, nursing programs need to create a culture of inclusion and belonging and recognize their achievements.

## Nurse Educator Pathways

There are nine themes that describe strategies for creating nurse educator pathways in the discussants' countries. The themes are Mentorship and Support, Faculty Development and Training, Financial Incentives and Compensation, Career Pathways and Advancement, Policy and Institutional Support, Visibility and Recruitment, Academic-Practice Partnerships, Curriculum and Teaching Innovation, and Workload and Flexibility.

### Mentorship and Support

An effective nurse educator pathway relies on strong mentorship. Mentoring needs to start with undergraduate nursing students who demonstrate promise for becoming future nursing faculty. Once hired as nursing faculty, senior faculty need to show support and mentor early-career faculty. Mentoring across all levels needs to outline pathways and include discussions about career advancement.

### *Faculty Development and Training*

Nursing faculty need regular training to remain effective, which starts with an intellectual humility of change. Training needs to start with a strong orientation program and/or faculty residency program, as well as be competency-based. Faculty development programs can be modeled after national programs, such as the Robert Wood Johnson Foundation Nurse Faculty Scholars and Moore Foundation programs. Nursing education should be recognized as a specialty practice of its own with a unique knowledge base and competencies. Nursing faculty development needs to focus on the science of nursing education. Nursing faculty also need to be cross-trained to teach in their specialty and in other types of courses.

### *Financial Incentives and Compensation*

For a nurse educator pathway to be effective in recruitment, the salary gap needs to be closed. Pay should be increased for nursing faculty, preceptors, and clinical instructors. Salary increases can be based on merit or retention incentives. Recruitment incentives can include more scholarships to full-time doctor of philosophy nursing students who commit to become faculty; increase loan forgiveness programs (e.g., U.S. Nurse Faculty Loan Program) for faculty and include preceptors and clinical instructors; and provide funds to support graduate assistantships to new faculty. Additional incentives include funds to support nursing faculty development, funds for formal mentoring and/or coaching, and teaching load release.

### *Career Pathways and Advancement*

A primary pathway is a "grow your own" approach where nursing faculty identify undergraduate students and mentor them to obtain their master of science degree and then to a full-time nurse faculty position. In addition, nursing faculty can provide opportunities for clinical nurses to be engaged in and exposed to teaching (e.g., become clinical preceptor). Once serving as a clinical preceptor, nurses can participate in a formal residency or preceptor-faculty accelerator pathway where they can teach a section of a course while advancing their degree to become eligible to be appointed as full-time faculty. Pathways need to provide mechanisms for regular promotion and leadership opportunities.

### *Policy and Institutional Support*

Institutions need to recognize teaching expertise as the same across all academic ranks and tracks (e.g., tenure track faculty teaching competency should be equivalent to a clinical educator teaching competency). Nursing programs can create a faculty development position (e.g., director of teaching) to ensure programs focus on effective teaching practices. Promotion policies should be clear but flexible based on track (e.g., clinical educator versus tenure). At a systems level, government policies should reflect the promotion and expansion of nurse educator pathways, requirements to become nursing faculty should be elevated, and sponsorship of statewide consortiums to support nursing faculty recruitment from doctoral programs is needed.

### *Visibility and Recruitment*

Nursing faculty need to change the narrative about being nursing faculty. This includes talking about the joys of academic nursing with students, promoting visibility of what a nurse faculty member is and does, and reframing the value of nursing faculty roles to be more inclusive of both clinical/education and research tracks. Recruitment activities can include engaging graduate nursing students and early-career nurses into nursing faculty career pathways, socializing doctor of philosophy students to find value in teaching, and having postdoctoral fellows teach one day per week. Formal campaigns need to be launched that publicize the role of nursing faculty and recognize the value of the nurse educator role.

### *Academic-Practice Partnerships*

A key strategy recommended by the discussants was to create academic-practice partnerships. These partnerships will allow for joint appointments of a nurse to be both a nurse faculty member and a clinician. An incentive program can be developed to encourage nurses to accept a joint appointment. New models of faculty practice need to be flexible and customizable based on the particular nurse, the teaching needs of the school, and the practice needs of the clinical agency.

### *Curriculum and Teaching Innovation*

Formal nurse educator programs are needed to create pathways for nurses to become academic faculty. Nursing programs can collaborate with clinical practice partners to design curriculum for future nursing faculty that will help them better teach the next generation of nurses to become faculty. Programs can terminate with a master of science degree or continue through to a doctoral degree. Schools can offer a minor or certificate program in nursing education for nurses matriculating in specialty master of science or doctor of nursing practice programs. Program components can include content about innovations in nursing education; resources for developing educational skills in AI, video lectures, and peer review; and opportunities to serve as a clinical preceptor. Nursing programs could strive to standardize their curriculum at the national level, offer their programs online and part-time, and collaborate to develop a Future Faculty Academy.

### *Workload and Flexibility*

Pathways for nurses to become nursing faculty need to accept that a manageable workload is an imperative. Nursing programs need to provide release time for nursing faculty to obtain a doctoral degree, learn their role, and attend professional development.

The workload needs to be flexible to allow release time when working on extramurally funded grant projects. In addition, workload needs to be balanced in the areas of teaching, scholarship, and service.

## Strategies to Promote Faculty Diversity

There are seven themes that describe strategies that can be used to promote diversity of the faculty in the discussants' countries. The themes are Recruitment Strategies, Mentorship and Career Development, Policy and Institutional Support, Inclusion and Culture, Community and Partnerships, Incentives and Funding, and Data and Evaluation.

### *Recruitment Strategies*

Formal recruitment is needed to promote a diverse faculty workforce. Recruitment strategies include formal campaigns, broad advertising, and inclusive recruitment practices. Inclusive recruitment practices were described as including diverse nurses in ads, placing ads in areas where they will be seen by diverse nurses, and expanding recruitment into a variety of settings and organizations. Discussants recommended several target populations from which to recruit to diversify the nursing faculty workforce: Indigenous nurses, LatinX nurses, male nurses, and nurses with disabilities. All nursing faculty should be engaged in recruitment activities. Nursing faculty could be purposeful in recruiting from within their networks: conduct targeted recruitment (e.g., "grow your own") and deliberate reach-out to colleagues working in clinical practice. Some discussants reported that not all faculty in nursing programs need to be nurses. There is a need to recruit and hire faculty from other disciplines, such as pharmacy, medicine, social work, and English. However, before nursing academia can become diverse, discussants emphasized that the general nursing workforce needs to diversify.

### *Mentorship and Career Development*

Nursing faculty should strategically recruit and mentor from a broad base of the nursing population to promote diversity in the faculty workforce. Nursing faculty can promote career development across multiple nursing entry points (e.g., licensed practical/vocational nurse to become a registered nurse to a nurse with a master of science degree; guest lecturer to full-time faculty). Early-career mentoring is needed for both those considering becoming nursing faculty and those novice to nursing education. Mentoring and career development also can include observing faculty in their role, implementing a visiting faculty program, having diverse faculty role models, and building supportive advisory groups to support nursing faculty and students.

### *Policy and Institutional Support*

Leadership should be committed to recruiting diverse faculty and set diversity as a priority for the nursing program and institution. Policies can be implemented such that, if all things are equal during the hiring phase, the underrepresented person should be hired (note that this may not be allowable in all countries). The organization should review all institutional policies and procedures for unintended barriers for promotion and potential bias. Position descriptions should be developed that allow a broad pool of faculty applicants. The position descriptions should clearly define teaching requirements. An additional policy can require faculty evaluations to occur every two to three years. The institution can further support nursing faculty diversity by promoting a positive workplace culture, ensuring leaders use authentic and transparent leadership, and promoting diverse faculty into leadership roles. At the policy level, governments can change laws to allow non-nationals to teach and practice in the country to which they immigrated, and accreditation requirements can require that faculty demographic composition represents the student population.

### *Inclusion and Culture*

Nursing programs need to create a welcoming environment, promote a culture of belonging, teach about cultural safety, celebrate differences, offer unconscious bias training, and quickly address signs or perceived signs of racism. Nursing faculty can host forums to discuss ideas about diversity and recognize the strengths of everyone. In addition, the definition of diversity needs to be broadened to be more inclusive.

### *Community and Partnerships*

Diversity of the nursing faculty workforce could be improved by partnering with clinical practice agencies. For example, underrepresented faculty from clinical sites can be recruited into a joint academic-practice appointment. Joint appointments also could be interprofessional and not specific to nurses. In addition, nursing programs can participate in nursing faculty exchange programs with other programs, schools, colleges, and/or universities to bring in underrepresented faculty. At a policy level, programs can advocate for state/provincial workforce development grants to include nursing education as a grant recipient to promote nursing faculty diversity.

### *Incentives and Funding*

Dedicated funding is needed to diversify the nursing faculty workforce. Funding should be provided for underrepresented nurses to pay for doctoral education (e.g., grants, scholarships) and incentives to become nursing faculty. Salary for underrepresented faculty should be equivalent to their peers. Additional resources should be offered to underrepresented faculty, such as approval for academic leave (e.g., sabbatical) and research awards, similar to what would be offered to other faculty members.

### *Data and Evaluation*

Data should be collected on the demographic characteristics of nursing faculty to determine if underrepresented faculty members are recruited and retained. These data can drive decision-making, and the findings should be shared widely. Formal research can be conducted to measure progress with recruitment and retention in addition to well-being issues for underrepresented faculty members.

# CONCLUSION

The nursing faculty shortage is a problem across multiple countries. Although the context of the nursing faculty shortage varies, the barriers to faculty recruitment were transferable across borders. Multi-component strategies are needed by individual faculty, nursing programs, clinical practice partners, and regulatory bodies to address nursing faculty recruitment challenges. Recruitment strategies need to be innovative to not only recruit enough nurses but also to recruit underrepresented nurses to become nursing faculty members. Mentoring, professional development, and equitable salary are key strategies needed to recruit and retain nursing faculty.

## *References*

Byrne, C., Keyt, J., & Fang, D. (2023, October). *Special survey on vacant faculty positions for academic year 2023–2024*. American Association of Colleges of Nursing. https://www.aacnnursing.org/Portals/0/PDFs/Data/Vacancy23.pdf

Calaguas, N. P. (2025). The role of co-teaching in strengthening nursing education amidst a global shortage. *Journal of Professional Nursing, 59*, 27–32. https://doi.org/10.1016/j.profnurs.2025.04.007

Christianson, J., Schindler, C., & Grabert, L. (2025). To address the nursing faculty shortage, start with the salary gap. *American Journal of Nursing, 125*(3), 8. https://doi.org/10.1097/AJN.0000000000000032

Fitzpatrick, K., & Forcina, J. (2026). Building academic-practice partnerships for clinical instructor partners: A step-by-step implementation framework. *Journal of Professional Nursing, 62*, 60–65. https://doi.org/10.1016/j.profnurs.2025.09.012

Gazza, E. A., Mehrlich, M., Earp, C. S., O'Brien, C., Balogh, P., & Stoffer, K. (2025). Expert clinician to novice educator using an academic nurse residency. *The Journal for Nurse Practitioners, 21*, 105280. https://doi.org/10.1016/j.nurpra.2024.105280

International Labour Office. (2005). *ILO nursing personnel convention no. 149.* International Labour Organization. https://www.ilo.org/publications/ilo-nursing-personnel-convention-no-149-recognize-their-contribution

Jones, C. B., Kim, S., Killela, M., Morgan, L., & Forcina, J. M. (2026). The transition, onboarding, and integration of newly hired faculty into nursing academia: A scoping review. *Journal of Professional Nursing, 62*, 66–82. https://doi.org/10.1016/j.profnurs.2025.10.010

Keenan, M. M., Kientz, E., Crossley, N. P., & Hoff, J. A. (2025). Practitioner-teacher model implementation within a newly integrated academic health system: Lessons learned. *Journal of Professional Nursing, 60*, 86–92. https://doi.org/10.1016/j.profnurs.2025.07.007

Kerns, C. J., & Wedgeworth, M. (2026). Increasing nursing faculty preparation through innovation in graduate and doctoral education. *Journal of Professional Nursing, 62*, 117–123. https://doi.org/10.1016/j.profnurs.2025.11.008

Sharpnack, P. A. (2025). Reflections on the global and national impact of the NLN: We do have the power to change the world. *Nursing Education Perspectives, 46*(5), 275. https://doi.org/10.1097/01.NEP.0000000000001456

PART 7

# Finding Hope in the Future

# 14

# Strategies and Confidence in the Future for Nursing Education at a Global Level

**Gordon Lee Gillespie, Sandra Davis, Teresa Shellenbarger, Ilse Wallace, Janice Brewington, Patricia A. Sharpnack, Larry Simmons, Kellie Bryant, Linda Christensen, Yolanda M. VanRiel, and Beverly Malone**

The NLN led an innovative and inaugural nursing-focused Utstein meeting. Nursing leaders and experts from 13 countries convened in Helsinki, Finland, in June 2025. The purpose of the NLN Utstein Conference on the Future of Nursing Education was to develop a vision for nursing education's future. The specific aims were to (1) list the priorities for the future of nursing education and (2) describe strategies, facilitators, and barriers for selected nursing education topics. We achieved our aims as evidenced in the previous chapters. This chapter provides a recap of the priorities for the future of nursing education; nine specific global recommendations; and implications for nursing education, nursing faculty, nursing programs, clinical practice, professional associations, and public policy based on Bronfenbrenner's (1977) social ecological model.

## PRIORITIES FOR THE FUTURE OF NURSING EDUCATION

As seen in Chapter 3, our predetermined focus areas of CBE, AI, planetary health, nurse and nursing faculty well-being, and global nursing faculty shortage were supported by discussants as priorities for the future of nursing education. Additional priorities also became prevalent. For example, technology inclusive of telehealth, simulation, and robotics as well as AI needs to be incorporated in future nursing curricula if students are to be better prepared to work in future health care systems. Also, leadership development needs to extend beyond what is offered today and focus on the executive leader preparing nurses to lead in the boardroom and in public-policy advocacy.

## GLOBAL RECOMMENDATIONS

Transforming nursing education is challenged by financial constraints, perceived lack of institutional commitment, limited infrastructure, perceived burdensome regulations and policies, the politicalization of higher education, rapid technology evolution including AI, a shortage of faculty experts, and a persistent global nursing faculty shortage. The lack of sufficient financial resources inhibits nursing programs from investing in technological innovations, closing the nursing faculty salary gap, hiring additional faculty, and supporting faculty development. With nursing education changing so rapidly, faculty face challenges maintaining their competence without adequate nursing faculty development and support. The lack of educational infrastructure could be partially driving the perceived lack of institutional commitment to advance nursing education. The academic work environment burdened by heavy workloads may be contributing to nursing faculty burnout, incivility, a lack of support, and the nursing faculty shortage. The following sections discuss recommendations to address the findings from the NLN Utstein Conference on the Future of Nursing Education.

## Recommendation 1: Nursing faculty need to be valued and recognized

The most pressing issue that prevents innovation and transformation for faculty is the lack of nursing faculty value and recognition of their work. One way to address this concern is to close the nursing faculty salary gap so that faculty salaries align with those of their clinical practice colleagues. In addition, nursing faculty need funds to support their professional development and enable nursing programs to contract with external experts to provide education and training on emerging topics (e.g., CBE, AI) and educational modalities (e.g., AR, simulation). Given the limited resources of many nursing programs, academic leaders may consider training a small group of nursing faculty to become experts who can then lead professional development within their own schools. In addition, many nursing faculty that are leading programs through innovative efforts, creative teaching, and learning approaches should be recommended for regional, national, and international awards, such as induction as a fellow into a national or international academy. Although some nursing faculty are making strides toward eligibility for these awards, they may need mentoring to fully achieve the award criteria. It is important to recognize that all nursing faculty need formal and informal mentoring, particularly those new to academic nursing.

## Recommendation 2: Nursing faculty workload needs to be achievable and equitable

Another priority is addressing nursing faculty workload. Discussants commonly reported that faculty workload was burdensome and limited their ability to achieve excellence in the tripartite mission of teaching, scholarship (e.g., research), and service. Some nursing faculty also have requirements to achieve excellence in clinical practice. As nursing faculty workload increases due to teaching overload, exacerbated by faculty shortage, nursing faculty have less time available to participate in faculty mentoring programs as a mentee and/or mentor; provide student mentoring; serve on or chair student projects and dissertations; seek extramural funding to support research and other scholarly efforts; and serve on committees at the school, university, and national levels. Nursing faculty need to partner with their program administrators to seek funding to hire enough faculty so that workload is equitably distributed. Financial support could be derived from school, college, and/or university reallocation of funds to the nursing program; new endowments for faculty positions; and private donations from health care systems, foundations, and industry sponsors.

## Recommendation 3: Competencies need to be standardized globally across nursing practice levels while allowing for cultural and contextual differences

Nursing education cannot be transformed into a globally standardized system until the nursing faculty shortage and workload are adequately addressed. Although agreement on common elements is important, nursing education also needs to accommodate the local and cultural contexts in which nursing programs are located. Standardization of nursing programs will require one or two associations with the capacity and skill to lead at a global level (e.g., NLN, ICN). These associations will require political prowess and consensus-building skills to manage the competing priorities of the requirements to enter the profession as a nurse. Minimum requirements vary not only across countries but also within countries (WHO, 2021). While some countries may require a formal college degree, other countries may license nurses at a practical/vocational level. Rather than focus exclusively on the minimum educational requirements to become a nurse, these association leaders can focus on the competencies and outcomes that need to be attained upon graduation to be ready to practice. The competencies and outcomes can be leveled across varying levels of practice (e.g., from practical/vocational nurse to doctorally prepared nurse). This focus will allow for seamless academic progression (Institute of Medicine, 2011). After this standardization occurs, nurses can more easily advance their education from entry level to advanced practice and doctoral levels and transition across clinical areas and countries.

A strategy emerging in the United States but more prevalent globally is CBE—a model of learning focused on achieving outcomes rather than passing courses and meeting a minimum number of hours in a clinical rotation (AACN/American Organization of Nurse Leaders [AONL] Academic-Practice Advisory Committee, 2025; NLN CBE Strategic Action Group, 2023). As CBE adoption takes place as recommended by the WHO (2021), competencies can more easily be standardized globally. Competency-based education, however, will require nursing programs to collaborate with their clinical practice partners, accrediting bodies, and boards of nursing to align competency expectations for their region, provide onsite clinical experiences to achieve those competencies, and avoid compliance risks. Collective accountability is necessary for clinical practice readiness.

## Recommendation 4: Nursing programs need to seek formal accreditation

All nursing programs should seek accreditation to demonstrate program quality (WHO, 2021). Formal program accreditation may be required to ensure that standardization of curricula occurs. A primary benefit of curricular standardization is that nurses can easily transition between nursing programs as they advance in their educational attainment. Achieving a specific level of practice competency would be recognized consistently across all nursing programs, thus preventing nursing students from needing to take additional courses to meet the new school's minimum entry requirements. Another benefit for nursing program applicants is the ability to be geographically mobile and choose a nursing program that aligns with their personal values, educational priorities, and ability to pay tuition. An example of personal values is applicants choosing a program based on a value of health care for all, with a programmatic focus on health equity and social determinants of health. In another example, applicants may choose a program based on its programmatic expertise, such as selecting a program internationally recognized for disaster nursing or another program recognized for family nurse practitioner education. Accreditation will require extensive faculty resources, training, and support, which may be challenging given the nursing faculty shortage and budgetary constraints (WHO, 2021).

## Recommendation 5: Nursing education should become specialized at the entry level

An innovation in nursing curricula is to move away from the generalist focus. Rather than preparing nursing students as generalists, as is often done in many countries, nursing students could specialize and focus on concentrated learning in a specialty area within their nursing program. Specialization already occurs within postlicensure graduate programs (e.g., public health clinical nurse specialist, nurse midwifery). This specialized education at the prelicensure level is used in Chamberlain University's (2026) "Practice Ready. Specialty Focused" program. Third-year students in the bachelor of science in nursing program are able to take additional coursework focused on one of five specialty tracks: emergency, home health, nephrology, perioperative, or oncology nursing. Afterward, students are immersed in an eight-week onsite clinical experience. Innovative specialty programs at the prelicensure level will allow students to adapt more quickly and be ready to practice in a nursing specialty after entering the profession as a licensed nurse. This could help shorten the time needed for graduate transition and allow nurse residency programs to have a more precise focus.

## Recommendation 6: Nursing programs need to embrace and incorporate technology/AI, planetary health, well-being, and executive leadership into their curricula

Nursing school curricula are notably congested with content intended to prepare graduates for every experience after graduation. Today's nursing curricula result from trying to address the evolving nature of health care while holding onto the past. Future nursing curricula need to prioritize content based on the future of health and health care. Advancements in technology, particularly through AI, are already radically changing health care. The incorporation of technology is necessary if nursing curricula are to remain relevant. Although technological advancements are becoming exponential, there are strategies that nursing programs can adopt. For example, nursing programs can use the same technologies used by their clinical partners. The clinical partners can provide software training accounts for nursing students to use the same software applications that they use. Students then can enter data to see the outputs (e.g., clinical practice recommendations) generated by technology (e.g., modified diet, screening for increased risk of renal insufficiency). As students increasingly use AI to complete assignments, guidelines are needed for the ethical use of AI (NLN AI Strategic Action Group, 2025). Faculty also can use AI to assist in generating and evaluating student assignments, thus potentially reducing faculty workload. AI can be leveraged by faculty and students for individualized learning, coaching, supporting, and tutoring.

Although planetary health may be a controversial topic in nursing (White et al., 2025), it remains a pressing global health concern. Without attention to planetary health in nursing curricula, students will be unable to advocate for and address problems related to disasters, climate change, and environmental toxins and waste. Nurses need to be prepared to educate "individuals, families, communities, and populations to address climate change strategies of mitigation, adaptation, and resilience" (NLN Climate Change and Health Strategic Action Group, 2022, p. 8). Nurses must educate their clients on disaster preparedness. Nurses also have a responsibility to examine their own behaviors and actions that contribute to climate change. They should work to reduce the waste created during routine clinical care. Reducing waste not only reduces toxins entering the environment but also lowers health care costs, making health care more affordable for all.

Nurses and nursing faculty continue to experience poor overall well-being. If well-being continues to be ignored in nursing curricula, the nursing profession will continue to lose its workforce. Well-being is essential to nursing curricula, should be embedded throughout programs, and should be based on local context and factors that impact the well-being of nurses and nursing faculty. The ICN writes that most national nurses' associations (86.2 percent) report that nurses experience workplace violence from patients, visitors, and coworkers (Sharplin et al., 2025). Students need training about workplace violence precursors, strategies to mitigate workplace violence, and how and when to seek support after incidents of workplace violence. Students need education to prepare them for the realities of their future roles and to address any mismatch with expectations and the stressors they may experience in clinical practice (e.g., workload, high-risk work, traumatic experiences, and low job control) (Sharplin et al., 2025). The curricula also can provide education on recognizing stress in oneself and obtaining support to manage this stress. Nursing faculty can role model well-being behaviors, such as maintaining a balance between work and personal responsibilities; interacting with students in relaxing, supportive settings; providing mentoring; and engaging in civil discourse (NLN Civil and Healthy Academic Work Environment Strategic Action Group, 2018). Of equal importance, nurses need to address their personal well-being in addition to that of their patients (White et al., 2025).

Nurses are increasingly being called to lead. This call to leadership goes beyond the typical executive skills of managing, supervising, and directing that nursing programs commonly prepare their graduates to perform. Nurses now need to be able to contribute to hospital boards, investigate opposing views on problems, provide expert recommendations, and make data-based executive decisions. Professional nurses add value to executive decision-making and contribute to these groups. For nurses to lead, they need executive leadership training to think strategically, persuade and influence others, inspire others to take action, and conduct critical evaluations of people and products (Robinson, 2024). Although not every nurse will secure a hospital board position, opportunities are available to serve on boards of local, state/provincial, and national government agencies; nonprofit organizations; and private companies. As people outside health care influence decision-making, nurses' leadership skills need to evolve. Now more than ever, nurses need to develop their ability to influence, inspire, and negotiate with policymakers, health care executives, and industry leaders.

## Recommendation 7: Nursing programs need to address the complexities of intersectionality, inclusion, equity, and social justice for the nursing profession

Nursing students, nurses, and nursing faculty are complex individuals composed of multiple identities. This intersectionality of identities can include their sex, gender, race, ability, educational attainment, citizenship, and other characteristics. Nursing programs need to acknowledge and accommodate these identities. For example, all newly licensed nurses may no longer need to be able to perform every skill that could be performed based on the highest level of clinical practice in an acute-care setting. As curricula are redesigned, faculty can ask whether every student who graduates needs to be able to independently perform all clinical skills. For example, does the graduate need to demonstrate manual chest compressions for resuscitation? This requirement excludes people with certain physical limitations from becoming or remaining a nurse. Physically performing chest compressions may no longer be required for all students, as technology and equipment involving mechanical compressive devices are now available to perform chest compressions. These devices have shown effectiveness in return of circulation and survival (Larik et al., 2024). However, nurses still need the competency to identify when chest compressions are warranted and to determine whether the technology/equipment is operating proficiently to achieve adequate perfusion during chest compressions. Another identity, such as race, was historically a factor prohibiting admission into nursing programs (Anchrum, 2025). Nursing programs can target recruitment efforts to underrepresented communities in their schools. Marketing strategies should be inclusive. Ultimately, a diverse workforce is needed to better provide culturally relevant care (Institute of Medicine, 2011).

Equity requires access to nursing programs for all. Because access can be particularly challenging for people in remote settings (e.g., rural, frontier area), nursing faculty and nursing schools need to invest in technology to ensure broader access for all students. Since the onset of the COVID-19 pandemic, many faculty learned to teach effectively in an online or via an e-learning environment (ICN, 2021). In addition to electronic instruction, AI might be leveraged to create simulation and VR experiences to augment clinical rotations and thus support learning in remote settings.

The content of nursing curricula also needs to evolve to address equity and social justice (White et al., 2025). Curricula need to link social determinants of health and health equity to a program's social mission, to address implicit and explicit bias, and to connect to health and wellness (NLN Social Determinants of Health Strategic Action Group, 2019). Clinical experiences can take place within clinical agencies that provide students with opportunities to address social determinants of health (NLN Social Determinants of Health Strategic Action Group, 2019). Nursing programs also need to ensure that students have broad clinical experiences. Clinical learning opportunities should not predominantly occur in a few acute-care settings. Students need exposure to communities in which they will practice. For example, students can be assigned clinical rotations to long-term care settings, public health departments, primary and secondary schools, and industry settings. Students also can complete a clinical learning rotation in a global setting, allowing them to experience a different health care system. These broad experiences will provide valuable skills and enable students to develop abilities such as recognizing the upstream and downstream impacts of health, equity, and justice in local, national, and global health care systems.

## Recommendation 8: Investments are needed into the development of the next generation of nursing faculty

With the ongoing global nursing faculty shortage, interventions are needed to increase and retain nursing faculty. Pipeline and career pathway programs can facilitate the transition of nurses into nursing faculty positions. Nurses can begin this transition by serving as clinical preceptors first, then moving into adjunct roles, and eventually full-time teaching roles. Formal advanced educational programs focused on preparing nurses for the scope of practice and competencies of academic nurse educators are needed to ensure adequately prepared nurses are ready for these faculty positions (Christensen & Simmons, 2026). Funding may be needed to support nurses' tuition and fees, as well as to provide the time required to complete these nurse educator programs.

Recruitment efforts of faculty into nursing programs need to consider that nursing education is a specialty nursing practice that should have minimum educational requirements to become a nurse educator, similar to nursing faculty credentialed to teach other advanced practice specialty programs (e.g., nurse anesthesia, nurse practitioner, nurse midwifery, clinical nurse specialist) (Christensen & Simmons, 2026; ICN, n.d.). Retention of nursing faculty will require several interventions, including closing the salary gap, offering supportive mentoring, addressing faculty workload, and providing ongoing professional development (ICN, n.d.).

To remain competent, nursing faculty need professional development on a range of topics, including instruction on using technology; revising curricula; incorporating and teaching CBE, AI, planetary health, nurse well-being, and executive leadership; evolving teaching modalities (e-learning, simulation, VR); and incorporating best practices in assessment, measurement, and evaluation. Professional development needs to ensure that faculty can demonstrate their expertise in these critical areas (WHO, 2021).

## Recommendation 9: An Institute for Research, Evaluation, Consultation, and Policy is needed to advance innovations in teaching and the science of nursing education

As evidenced in this report, faculty and nursing programs across the globe need evidence to support nursing teaching practices. Although the findings in this report are based on the cumulative knowledge and expertise of nurse scholars from 13 countries, additional evidence is needed to support these conclusions and evaluate the effectiveness of these changes. Therefore, significant advancement is needed for the science of nursing education. A key strategy requires the creation of an Institute for Research, Evaluation, Consultation, and Policy. This institute could:

- Employ a cadre of nurse scientists building the science of nursing education.
- Provide research grants to nurse scientists focused on the science of nursing education.
- Become a global hub for experts focused on advancing the future of nursing education, CBE, AI and other technologies, planetary health, nurse and nursing faculty well-being, executive leadership, and the workforce.
- Provide consultation and evaluation services to nursing programs worldwide.
- Write public policy recommendations and white papers related to nursing education.
- Influence government, legislation, and public-policy rulemaking on nursing education.
- Develop a repository of resources focused on research designs, data collection instruments, and methods to support the advancement of the science of nursing education, grantsmanship, effective evaluations, accreditation, public policymaking, and professional development.
- Offer professional development on effective teaching, learning, and evaluation practices.
- Provide formal mentoring to faculty and nurses wanting to become nursing faculty.

# IMPLICATIONS

This section provides a list of actionable implementation strategies to move the recommendations beyond vision and into action (see Table 14.1). Recommendations or strategies are organized by level of intervention (faculty/nurse educator; program, school, college, and university; national; international) in alignment with Bronfenbrenner's (1977) social ecological model. Recommendations or strategies are further categorized based on a focus of nursing education, nursing faculty, nursing programs, clinical practice, professional associations, and public policy.

**TABLE 14.1**

## Recommendations/Strategies for the Future of Nursing Education

| Level of Intervention | Recommendation/Strategy |
|---|---|
| Faculty/Nurse Educator (microsystem) | **Focus on nursing education:**<br>➤ Educate students to be ready to practice<br>➤ Engage students as partners in their education<br>➤ Incorporate active teaching and learning strategies (e.g., gaming) that engage students in their learning<br>➤ Incorporate executive leadership development across curricula<br>➤ Use a competency-based framework to conduct a curriculum and assessment crosswalk to transition to CBE (NLN CBE Strategic Action Group, 2023)<br>➤ Develop/review policies, resources, and practices to support personalized learning and course progression (e.g., assessment retake policies, prior learning) (NLN CBE Strategic Action Group, 2023)<br>➤ Redesign curricula to embed AI content in clinical reasoning, simulation, informatics, and ethics courses (NLN AI Strategic Action Group, 2025)<br>➤ Use AI-enhanced learning tools (e.g., virtual avatars, predictive analytics) to personalize instruction (NLN AI Strategic Action Group, 2025)<br>➤ Leverage technology to track competency attainment<br>➤ Establish clear policies and guidelines for AI integration into nursing programs<br>**Focus on nursing faculty:**<br>➤ Model responsible AI use, emphasizing human oversight and critical thinking (NLN AI Strategic Action Group, 2025)<br>➤ Model self-care and professional well-being (e.g., stress management, building resiliency) for faculty, recognizing the importance of looking at self before leading others (NLN Civil and Healthy Academic Work Environment Strategic Action Group, 2018)<br>**Focus on clinical practice:**<br>➤ Collaborate with clinical practice partners to identify and verify key competencies for contemporary clinical practice (NLN CBE Strategic Action Group, 2023)<br>➤ Co-develop curriculum with clinical partners (AACN/AONL Academic-Practice Advisory Committee, 2025)<br>➤ Share data and tools to train students on real-world AI platforms used in clinical settings (NLN AI Strategic Action Group, 2025)<br>➤ Co-create simulation and clinical learning experiences that incorporate AI-based decision-making tools (NLN AI Strategic Action Group, 2025) |

(*continued*)

**TABLE 14.1**

**Recommendations/Strategies for the Future of Nursing Education** (*continued*)

| Level of Intervention | Recommendation/Strategy |
|---|---|
| | **Focus on public policy:**<br>➤ Advance educational strategies to ensure that students learn policy and advocacy skills, specifically addressing health consequences of climate change, to communicate with policymakers at local, state, national, international, and global levels (NLN Climate Change and Health Strategic Action Group, 2022)<br>➤ Develop community partnerships for students to work with local communities to address impacts of climate change and health (NLN Climate Change and Health Strategic Action Group, 2022)<br>➤ Advocate for fair and equitable recovery for individuals and communities after wildfires, hurricanes, floods, and other destructive climate-related events to decrease the need for downstream health care responses (NLN Climate Change and Health Strategic Action Group, 2022) |
| Program, School, College, and University (mesosystem) | **Focus on nursing education:**<br>➤ Adopt technology to track student competency attainment<br>➤ Provide specialization of practice while in nursing schools<br>➤ Adopt or expand interprofessional education<br>➤ Offer microcredentials or graduate programs focused on nursing education<br>➤ Develop partnerships with other programs and disciplines in elevating the recognition and value of nursing with the greater academic system<br>**Focus on nursing faculty:**<br>➤ Focus on faculty development<br>➤ Provide leadership development to faculty and academic leaders<br>**Focus on nursing programs:**<br>➤ Facilitate clear communication and transparency of competency outcomes with all interested parties, including students and clinical practice partners (NLN CBE Strategic Action Group, 2023)<br>➤ Establish an AI governance and oversight committee within nursing schools (NLN AI Strategic Action Group, 2025)<br>➤ Strengthen partnerships with health care systems and AI industry to promote collaborative learning environment for learners (NLN AI Strategic Action Group, 2025)<br>➤ Share resources with other nursing programs to reduce individual program burden and financial impact |

**TABLE 14.1**

**Recommendations/Strategies for the Future of Nursing Education** (*continued*)

| Level of Intervention | Recommendation/Strategy |
|---|---|
| National (exosystem) | **Focus on clinical practice:**<br>➤ Recognize that newly licensed nurses will continue to need support and ongoing training and development after hire (AACN/AONL Academic-Practice Advisory Committee, 2025)<br>➤ Develop policies to ensure balance between enhancing technology while not replacing nurses with technology<br>**Focus on professional associations:**<br>➤ Develop additional Centers of Excellence programs for selected topics (e.g., AI)<br>**Focus on public policy:**<br>➤ Invest in information technology and equipment to increase access to digital technology for students and faculty in remote areas (WHO, 2021) |
| International (macrosystem) | **Focus on professional associations:**<br>➤ Develop a network of nursing faculty and scientists to participate in international nursing faculty exchange programs to build research capacity globally (WHO, 2021)<br>**Focus on public policy:**<br>➤ Collaborate with clinical practice partners and national and international organizations to promote the adoption of CBE (NLN CBE Strategic Action Group, 2023)<br>➤ Implement multi-national programs focused on celebrating nurses throughout the year including motivational and team-building activities and employee health and wellness programs (Gulf Health Council, 2025)<br>➤ Promote and encourage the work of the ICN Education Experts Advisory Committee<br>➤ Ensure compliance with the WHO Global Code of Practice on the International Recruitment of Health Personnel (WHO, 2021) |

## CONCLUSION

The NLN Utstein Conference on the Future of Nursing Education was a highly successful meeting generating thousands of recommendations for nursing education. These recommendations, summarized in this report, provide a guidebook or map for revolutionizing and transforming nursing curricula worldwide. By adopting and/or customizing the recommendations in this report, particularly those in this chapter, nursing faculty can lead curricular redesign, incorporate innovative teaching modalities, and embed forward-thinking topics to ensure the next generation of nursing graduates is ready to enter clinical practice. Future Utstein meetings can build on these results by focusing on select topics that continue to advance the science of nursing education while building greater consensus across more nursing experts and national nursing associations.

## References


AACN/AONL Academic-practice Advisory Committee. (2025, November). *The AACN/AONL academic-practice partnership playbook: From shared vision to action*. American Organization for Nursing Leadership. https://www.aonl.org/system/files/media/file/2025/11/AACN-AONL-Academic-Practice-Partnership-Playbook.pdf

Anchrum, H. (2025). Through the eyes of Black nurses: The impact of the Nurse Training Act of 1964. *Policy, Politics, & Nursing Practice*, *26*(1), 56–64. https://doi.org/10.1177/15271544241296825

Bronfenbrenner, U. (1977). Toward an experimental ecology of human development. *American Psychologist, 32*(7), 513–531. https://doi.org/10.1037/0003-066X.32.7.513

Chamberlain University. (2026). *Practice ready. Specialty focused*. Chamberlain University. https://www.chamberlain.edu/practice-ready-specialty-focused

Christensen, L. S., & Simmons, L. E. (2026). *The scope of practice for academic nurse educators practicing in various academic nurse educator roles* (4th ed.). NLN Press.

Gulf Health Council. (2025, May). *Annual report 2024*. Gulf Health Council. https://www.ghc.sa/wp-content/uploads/2025/05/Gulf-Health-Annual-Report-2024-1.pdf

Institute of Medicine. (2011). *The future of nursing: Leading change, advancing health*. The National Academies Press.

International Council of Nursing. (2021, April). *International Council of Nurses policy brief: Nursing education and the emerging nursing workforce in COVID-19 pandemic*. International Council of Nursing. https://www.icn.ch/sites/default/files/2023-04/ICN%20Policy%20Brief_Nursing%20Education.pdf

Larik, M. O., Ahmed, A., Shiraz, M. I., Shiraz, S. A., Anjum, M. U., & Bhattarai, P. (2024). Comparison of manual chest compression versus mechanical chest compression for out-of-hospital cardiac arrest: A systematic review and meta-analysis. *Medicine*, *103*, 8. http://dx.doi.org/10.1097/MD.0000000000037294

National League for Nursing Artificial Intelligence Strategic Action Group. (2025, September). *NLN vision statement: Artificial intelligence (AI) in nursing education*. National League for Nursing. https://www.nln.org/docs/default-source/default-document-library/nln_ai_vision_statement.pdf?sfvrsn=dbb7bef_1

National League for Nursing Civil and Healthy Academic Work Environment Strategic Action Group. (2018, September). *NLN vision statement: Creating community to build a civil and healthy academic work environment*. National League for Nursing. https://www.nln.org/docs/default-source/uploaded-files/professional-development-programs/vision-statement-a-vision-for-creating-community-to-build-a-civil-and-healthy.pdf?sfvrsn=2ca7ab0d_0&pdf=VisionSeries-CreatingCommunity

National League for Nursing Climate Change and Health Strategic Action Group. (2022, September). *NLN vision statement: Climate change and health*. National League for Nursing. https://www.nln.org/docs/default-source/default-document-library/vision-series-climate-change-health.pdf?sfvrsn=86ee3340_3

National League for Nursing Competency-Based Education Strategic Action Group. (2023, January). *NLN vision statement: Integrating competency-based education in the nursing curriculum*. National League for Nursing. https://www.nln.org/docs/default-source/default-document-library/vision-series_integrating-competency-based-education-in-the-nursing-curriculum-d6eb0a1e-1f8b-4d60-bc4f-619f5e75b445.pdf?sfvrsn=b37e7538_3

National League for Nursing Social Determinants of Health Strategic Action Group.

(2019, April). *NLN vision statement: A vision for integration of the social determinants of health into nursing education curricula*. National League for Nursing. https://www.nln.org/docs/default-source/default-document-library/social-determinants-of-health.pdf?sfvrsn=6078db72_1

Robinson, S. (2024, August 16). *What is executive leadership?* TechTarget. https://www.techtarget.com/searchcio/definition/executive-leadership

Sharplin, G., Clarke, J., & Eckert, M. (2025, March). *Assessing the global sustainability of the nursing workforce a survey of national nurses' association presidents within the international council of nurses.* International Council of Nurses. https://www.icn.ch/sites/default/files/2025-04/ICN_NNA-Presidents-Survey-Report_EN_FINAL.pdf

White, J., Gunn, M., Chiarella, M., Catton, H., & Stewart, D. (2025, June). *Renewing the definitions of 'nursing' and 'a nurse': Final project report, June 2025*. International Council of Nurses. https://www.icn.ch/sites/default/files/2025-06/ICN_Definition-Nursing_Report_EN_Web_0.pdf

World Health Organization. (2021). *Global strategic directions for nursing and midwifery: 2021-2025.* World Health Organization. https://iris.who.int/server/api/core/bitstreams/11723bae-3fd4-46f0-a4ea-9dc8fd153667/content

# Appendix

# Roster of World Café Leaders, Table Hosts, and Discussants

## WORLD CAFÉ LEADERS

- **Sandra DAVIS**, PhD, DPM, ACNP-BC, FAANP, FAAN, Deputy Chief Director, National League for Nursing, United States, REGION OF THE AMERICAS
- **Gordon Lee GILLESPIE**, PhD, DNP, RN, CEN, CNE, CPEN, PHCNS-BC, ANEF, FAEN, FAAN, Chief Program Officer, National League for Nursing, United States, REGION OF THE AMERICAS

## WORLD CAFÉ TABLE HOSTS

- **Janice G. BREWINGTON**, PhD, RN, FADLN, FAAN, Consultant and Retired Director, Center for Transformational Leadership, National League for Nursing, United States, REGION OF THE AMERICAS
- **Kellie BRYANT**, DNP, WHNP, FSSH, FADLN, FAAN, Director of the Center for Innovation in Education Excellence, National League for Nursing, United States, REGION OF THE AMERICAS
- **Linda CHRISTENSEN**, EdD, JD, RN, FAAN, Chief Legal Officer, National League for Nursing, United States, REGION OF THE AMERICAS
- **Patricia SHARPNACK**, DNP, RN, CNE, NEA-BC, ANEF, FAAN, Dean and Strawbridge Professor, The Breen School of Nursing and Health Professions, Ursuline College and Immediate Past Chair, National League for Nursing, United States, REGION OF THE AMERICAS
- **Teresa SHELLENBARGER**, PhD, RN, CNE, CNEcl, ANEF, FAAN, Executive Director, National League for Nursing Commission for Nursing Education Accreditation, United States, REGION OF THE AMERICAS
- **Larry SIMMONS**, PhD, RN, CNE, CGNC, ICE-CCP, FAAN, Senior Director of Credentialing (Retired), National League for Nursing, United States, REGION OF THE AMERICAS
- **Deborah TRAUTMAN**, PhD, RN, FAAN, President and Chief Executive Officer, American Association of Colleges of Nursing, United States, REGION OF THE AMERICAS

- **Yolanda VANRIEL**, PhD, RN, MEDSURG-BC, OCN, CNE, ANEF, Nursing Department Chair, North Carolina Central University and Chair, Board of Governors, National League for Nursing, United States, REGION OF THE AMERICAS
- **Ilse WALLACE**, PhD, RN, CNE, Executive Dean, Academic Quality, Chamberlain University, United States, REGION OF THE AMERICAS

## WORLD CAFÉ DISCUSSANTS

- **Laila Mahmoud AKHU-ZAHEYA**, PhD, RN, Dean and Professor, Jordan University of Science and Technology, Jordan, EASTERN MEDITERRANEAN REGION
- **Naeema AL QASSEER**, PhD, RN, RM, FAAN, Advisory Board Member at Qatar University Health Cluster Bahrain Nursing & Midwifery Association Advisor, Kingdom of Bahrain, EASTERN MEDITERRANEAN REGION
- **Salem Said AL TOUBY**, PhD, Dean and Associate Professor, College of Health Sciences, University of Nizwa, Oman, EASTERN MEDITERRANEAN REGION
- **Maryann ALEXANDER**, PhD, RN, FAAN, Visiting Professor, Vanderbilt University, United States, REGION OF THE AMERICAS
- **Angela F. AMAR**, PhD, RN, ANEF, FAAN, Dean & Professor, New York University Rory Meyers College of Nursing, United States, REGION OF THE AMERICAS
- **Lydia AZIATO**, PhD, MPhil, FWACN, FASLP, FGCNM, BA, Vice-Chancellor, University of Health and Allied Sciences, Ghana, AFRICAN REGION
- **Ryan BARRETT**, RN, President, National Student Nurses' Association, United States, REGION OF THE AMERICAS
- **Anne R. BAVIER**, PhD, RN, FAAN, NLN President 2015–2017 and Professor Emeritus, University of Texas at Arlington, United States, REGION OF THE AMERICAS
- **Ann BONNER**, PhD, MA, BAppSc, RN, MACN, MAICD, Professor, Griffith University, Australia, WESTERN PACIFIC REGION
- **Katie BOSTON-LEARY**, PhD, MBS, MHA, RN, NEA-BC, FADLN, FAONL, Senior Vice President of Equity and Engagement, American Nurses Enterprise, United States, REGION OF THE AMERICAS
- **Latina BROOKS**, PhD, APRN, FAANP, Associate Professor and Assistant Dean of Graduate & Professional Programs, Case Western Reserve University, United States, REGION OF THE AMERICAS
- **Jacquelyn CAMPBELL**, PhD, RN, FAAN, Professor, Johns Hopkins University School of Nursing, United States, REGION OF THE AMERICAS
- **Kathy CHAPPELL**, PhD, RN, FNAP, FAAN, Chief Executive Officer, Accreditation Commission for Education in Nursing, United States, REGION OF THE AMERICAS
- **Earl DALTON**, MHS, MSL, RN, NEA-BC, FAAN, Chief Clinical Officer & VP Clinical Services, Health Carousel, United States, REGION OF THE AMERICAS

- **Nuhad Yazbkik DUMIT**, RN, MA, PhD, Professor, American University of Beirut, Lebanon, EASTERN MEDITERRANEAN REGION
- **Joyce FITZPATRICK**, PhD, MBA, RN, FAAN, FNAP, FAANP(H), Director, Marian K. Shaughnessy Nurse Leadership Academy, Francis Payne Bolton School of Nursing, Case Western Reserve University, United States, REGION OF THE AMERICAS
- **Cristina GARCÍA-VIVAR**, PhD, MSc, Professor of Nursing, Public University of Navarre, Spain, EUROPEAN REGION
- **Rakhi GAUR**, PhD, RN, Assistant Professor, College of Nursing, All India Institute of Medical Sciences, India, SOUTH-EAST ASIA REGION
- **Jean GIDDENS**, PhD, RN, FAAN, ANEF, Professor and Dean, University of Kansas School of Nursing and Chair, Board of Directors, American Association of Colleges of Nursing, United States, REGION OF THE AMERICAS
- **Pandora HARDTMAN**, DNP, CNM, RN, FACNM, FAAN, Chief Nursing & Midwifery Officer, Jhpiego, Bermuda, REGION OF THE AMERICAS
- **Michelle HEREFORD**, MSHA, RN, FACHE, Chief Nurse Executive, University Hospitals Health System, United States, REGION OF THE AMERICAS
- **Pamela JEFFRIES**, PhD, RN, FAAN, ANEF, FSSH, Dean and Valere Potter Distinguished Professor, Vanderbilt University School of Nursing, United States, REGION OF THE AMERICAS
- **Jan JONES-SCHENK**, DHSc, RN, FAADN, FAAN, Executive Dean Emeritus, Leavitt School of Health, Western Governors University, United States, REGION OF THE AMERICAS
- **Paule Valery JOSEPH**, PhD, MBA, MS, FNP-BC, CTN-B, FAAN, Lasker Clinical Research Investigator and Co-director of the National Smell and Taste Center, National Institutes of Health, United States, REGION OF THE AMERICAS
- **Sook Jung KANG**, PhD, FNP-C, Associate Professor, College of Nursing, Ewha Woman's University, South Korea, WESTERN PACIFIC REGION
- **Amy KLINE**, MA, RN, CHSE, Head of Competency Based Education, Laerdal Medical, United States, REGION OF THE AMERICAS
- **Sami LAMA**, MSc Nursing, RN, Professor, College of Nursing, B.P. Koirala Institute of Health Sciences, Nepal, WESTERN PACIFIC REGION
- **Karine LAVOIE**, MSc, MSN, RN, CWOCN, CHSE, PMP, Head of Education, Partnerships and Programme Development, International Council of Nursing, Switzerland, EUROPEAN REGION
- **Rhonda LAWES**, PhD, RN, Chief Nursing Officer, Lecturio, United States, REGION OF THE AMERICAS
- **Andrea LINDELL**, RN, BSN, MSN, PhD, ANEF, Dean Emerita and Former Vice-Provost for Social Determinants of Health and Advancement, College of Nursing, Walden University, United States, REGION OF THE AMERICAS
- **Andrew LINGO**, Director-Ethical Recruitment & Sustainability, Health Carousel, United States, REGION OF THE AMERICAS

- **Beverly MALONE**, PhD, RN, FAAN, President and Chief Executive Officer, National League for Nursing, United States, REGION OF THE AMERICAS
- **Yolanda OGBOLU**, PhD, RN, NNP, FNAP, FAAN, Bill and Joanne Conway Dean and Professor, University of Maryland School of Nursing, United States, REGION OF THE AMERICAS
- **Tracy A. ORTELLI**, PhD, RN, CNE, ANEF, FAAN, President & Chief Academic Officer, Galen College of Nursing, United States, REGION OF THE AMERICAS
- **Christine PABICO**, PhD, RN, NE-BC, FAAN, FFNMRCSI, Sr. Director, Pathway to Excellence and Well-Being Excellence, American Nurses Credentialing Center, United States, REGION OF THE AMERICAS
- **Teddie POTTER**, PhD, RN, FAAN, FNAP, Clinical Professor and Director, Center for Planetary Health and Environmental Justice, School of Nursing, University of Minnesota, United States, REGION OF THE AMERICAS
- **Peter PREZIOSI**, PhD, RN, CAE, President & Chief Executive Officer, TruMerit, United States, REGION OF THE AMERICAS
- **Anne Marie RAFFERTY**, PhD, RN, Baroness and Professor, King's College, United Kingdom, EUROPEAN REGION
- **Elizabeth REYNA**, CAE, Membership Director and Foundation Manager, National League for Nursing, United States, REGION OF THE AMERICAS
- **F. Patrick ROBINSON**, PhD, RN, ACRN, CNE, ANEF, FAAN, Vice President of Nursing, Pacific College of Health and Science, United States, REGION OF THE AMERICAS
- **Cynda Hylton RUSHTON**, PhD, RN, FAAN, Anne & George Bunting Professor of Clinical Ethics and Professor of Nursing and Pediatrics, Johns Hopkins University, United States, REGION OF THE AMERICAS
- **Suresh SHARMA**, PhD, RN, FNRS, FAAN, Professor and Principal, College of Nursing, All India Institute of Medical Sciences, India, SOUTH-EAST ASIA REGION
- **Mikhail SHNEYDER**, DNEd(hc), MBA, RN, Chief Executive Officer, Nightingale Education Group, United States, REGION OF THE AMERICAS
- **Erin SLAY**, DNP, MHA, RN, Associate Dean, Central School of Practical Nursing, United States, REGION OF THE AMERICAS
- **Suzanne C. SMELTZER**, EdD, RN, ANEF, FAAN, Professor Emerita and Adjunct Faculty, M. Louise Firtzpatrick College of Nursing, Villanova University, United States, REGION OF THE AMERICAS
- **Erin SNELGROVE-CLARKE**, PhD, Professor, School of Nursing, Faculty of Health Sciences, Queen's University, Canada, REGION OF THE AMERICAS
- **Maxim TOPAZ**, PhD, RN, FAAN, FACMI, FIAHSI, Elizabeth Standish Gill Associate Professor, Columbia University, United States, REGION OF THE AMERICAS
- **Josefa VASQUEZ CEVALLOS**, PhD, MS, RN, National Dean, College of Nursing of Perú, Perú, REGION OF THE AMERICAS

- **Antonia M. VILLARRUEL**, PhD, RN, FAAN, Professor and Margaret Bond Simon Dean of Nursing, University of Pennsylvania, United States, REGION OF THE AMERICAS
- **Kenya WILLIAMS**, EdD, MBA, MSN, RN, RP, CAE, FNYAM, FADNL, FAAN, Chief Executive Officer, National Student Nurses' Association, United States, REGION OF THE AMERICAS
- **Patricia S. YODER-WISE**, EdD, RN, NEA-BC, ANEF, FAONL, FAAN, President and Dean Emerita, Texas Tech University Health Sciences Center, United States, REGION OF THE AMERICAS